T0222172

KEY TRIALS IN INTENSIVE CARE MEDICINE

This essential guide encompasses over 160 pivotal papers critical for doctors preparing for postgraduate exams in intensive care, interviews, or commencing an intensive care rotation. Chosen for their educational merit and significant influence on intensive care medicine, these key trials, studies, and meta-analyses are distilled into succinct, easy-to-read summaries.

The guide steers clear of intricate numerical details and statistical analyses, concentrating instead on the core information necessary to comprehend the significance of these influential papers. Tailored specifically for the OSCE and SOE components of exams like the Final FFICM and EDIC, it provides concise summaries and key results, focusing on the most crucial information for exam success.

Serving as a resource that underpins the evidence base of contemporary intensive care clinical practice, these summaries are an indispensable tool for both exam preparation and ongoing professional development in intensive care medicine.

KEY TRIALS IN INTENSIVE CARE MEDICINE

PASSING THE FINAL FFICM

Muzzammil Ali and Joanna Kondratowicz

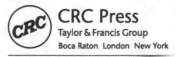

CRC Press

Taylor & Francis Group
Boca Raton London New York

CRC Press is an imprint of the
Taylor & Francis Group, an **informa** business

First edition published 2025
by CRC Press
4 Park Square, Milton Park, Abingdon, Oxon, OX14 4RN

and by CRC Press
2385 NW Executive Center Drive, Suite 320, Boca Raton, FL 33431

CRC Press is an imprint of Informa UK Limited

ISBN: 978-1-032-74329-5 (hbk)
ISBN: 978-1-032-74327-1 (pbk)
ISBN: 978-1-003-46873-8 (ebk)

DOI: 10.1201/9781003468738

Typeset in Times
by Apex CoVantage, LLC

*Dedicated to all aspiring intensivists pursuing
excellence in intensive care medicine.*

*With warm hearts, we also dedicate this to Joanna's parents,
George and Ewa, her sister Monika, and to Muzzammil's
parents, Nizam and Amina, and his sister Nura. Your
unwavering support and love are our constant inspiration.*

*Additionally, we extend this dedication to our
esteemed colleagues, whose invaluable mentorship,
constant encouragement, and nurturing environment
have been instrumental in our growth.*

Contents

Foreword

Research in intensive care medicine has expanded exponentially in recent years, with many key trials changing practice. Keeping up to date with the latest evidence is a challenging but essential task for any clinician, especially those undertaking exams. The Fellowship of the Faculty of Intensive Care Medicine examination ensures that future intensive care consultants are assessed and perform to a high standard. Understanding the evidence base underpinning practice is key in preparing for this examination.

Key Trials in Intensive Care Medicine is an indispensable resource for efficient exam preparation for the FFICM oral examination. This book provides an up-to-date summary of key trials, organised by time and subject in a way that is easy to digest and recall in an exam setting. It summarises the evidence base through key trials across the entirety of the intensive care curriculum and is pitched at the right level of detail for the FFICM examination.

The authors have a proven track record in medical education. They not only excel in exams themselves but have also assisted colleagues in navigating the challenging oral section of the FFICM. With this useful resource, I have no doubt many others will benefit.

Dr Mohammed Asif Arshad
MB, BChir, MRCP, FRCA, FFICM, MA (Pharm),
MSc (Hcl), PGCME
Consultant in Anaesthesia and Intensive Care Medicine
University Hospitals Birmingham NHS Foundation Trust
West Midlands Trainee Programme Director for
Intensive Care Medicine

Preface

We are delighted to present *Key Trials in Intensive Care Medicine*, a guide developed for candidates preparing for the Final FFICM or equivalent exams. This book encompasses over 160 pivotal trials, studies, or meta-analyses, each selected for its lasting impact and educational value in intensive care medicine.

Recognising the need for a consolidated resource summarising key trials for the Final FFICM exam, we have meticulously crafted this guide. It is designed to equip candidates with robust, evidence-based information, particularly focusing on the OSCE and SOE components of the exam. The aim is to assist in answering the crucial question, 'What is the evidence for . . .?' and lays a strong foundation for both exam success and ongoing professional discussions.

Organised by organ system and arranged thematically based on the year of publication, this book presents each trial in a concise table format. These tables summarise the study population, intervention, and primary and secondary outcomes and include a 'viva summary'—a brief overview for exam viva scenarios—for quick reference. The 'Study Conclusion' directly quotes the researchers' original findings, adding depth and context. References for further reading are provided below each summary.

To support efficient revision, particularly in the final stages of exam preparation, each chapter concludes with a 'Summary,' compiling all viva summaries for easy reference. This guide, intended for use alongside primary study materials, offers a comprehensive review of study outcomes, consciously avoiding numerical details and statistical analysis. In some cases, less critical study details not essential for the exam have been omitted.

The fundamental purpose of this book, therefore, is to facilitate the quick recall of the most salient findings from these trials. It is designed not to delve into a deep critique of these trials, such as the analysis of confounding factors or interpretation of results and their clinical implications, but rather to underscore the statistical significance of findings without exploring their extent. Although some of the included trials may be less current, their inclusion is crucial for providing comprehensive and relevant responses in the exam setting and for understanding the evolution of ICU practices.

We extend our best wishes for your success in your FFICM journey and encourage you to explore our companion book, *Passing the Final FFICM: High-Yield Facts for the MCQ & OSCE Exams*, for additional preparation.

Muzzammil Ali
Joanna Kondratowicz

Authors

Dr Muzzammil Ali, a graduate of the University of Birmingham, UK, is a Senior Registrar in Intensive Care and Acute Internal Medicine in the West Midlands. He successfully completed the Final FFICM exam in April 2022. Dedicated to medical education, he focuses on assisting trainees to excel in medical exams and achieve ultrasound accreditation. Muzzammil holds leadership roles at Queen Elizabeth Hospital Birmingham, serves as an Honorary Clinical Lecturer at the University of Birmingham, and represents West Midlands trainees in Intensive Care Medicine.

Dr Joanna Kondratowicz, a medical graduate from the University of Bristol, UK, also holds a First-Class intercalated degree in bioethics. She currently works as an Internal Medicine Trainee in London, UK, and has successfully completed her MRCP(UK) postgraduate exams. Kondratowicz's keen interest in Intensive Care Medicine was sparked during her redeployment to critical care amidst the COVID-19 pandemic, and she has since continued to gain experience in this exciting specialty.

Disclaimer

- *Scope and educational purpose*: This guide is specifically tailored for medical professionals preparing for the Final FFICM or similar examinations. It highlights key themes and concepts vital for SOE/OSCE responses. Not all trials pertinent to intensive care medicine are included in this guide. Instead, it offers a curated selection of the most cited trials, streamlined for study without exhaustive detail, based on feedback and citations from peers, textbooks, and conferences. It prioritises key insights over comprehensive statistical analysis or critical appraisal. Unless specified otherwise, trials predominantly involve adult subjects.

- *Clinical relevance*: This educational resource is designed for exam preparation rather than direct clinical application, emphasising insights critical for exam success. It selectively covers content, omitting less crucial details to enhance revision effectiveness. While providing a basic understanding, readers should consult original studies for deeper insights and assess their applicability to contemporary clinical settings.

- *Relevance and updates*: Trials included in this guide are selected for their lasting educational value, even if some are dated. They are intended to support thorough exam responses and should be considered in light of ongoing developments in clinical practice. Readers are encouraged to evaluate both the historical and present relevance of these trials in their application to practice.

Abbreviations

AAA	Abdominal Aortic Aneurysm
ACLS	Advanced Cardiac Life Support
AF	Atrial Fibrillation
AIS	Abbreviated Injury Scale
AKI	Acute Kidney Injury
ALS	Advanced Life Support
AP	Acute Pancreatitis
ARDS	Acute Respiratory Distress Syndrome
ATN	Acute Tubular Necrosis
BDG	(1,3)-β-D-Glucan
BMES	Balanced Multielectrolyte Solution
CI	Confidence Interval
CPC	Cerebral Performance Category
CRBSI	Catheter-Related Bloodstream Infection
CVC	Central Venous Catheter
CVVHDF	Continuous Veno-Venous Haemodiafiltration
DCI	Delayed Cerebral Ischaemia
DL	Direct Laryngoscope
$ECCO_2R$	Extracorporeal Carbon Dioxide Removal
ECMO	Extracorporeal Membrane Oxygenation
ECPR	Extracorporeal Cardiopulmonary Resuscitation
ED	Emergency Department
EGDT	Early Goal-Directed Therapy
EVAR	Endovascular Aneurysm Repair
FEV_1	Forced Expiratory Volume in the first second
FiO_2	Fraction of inspired Oxygen
FFP	Fresh Frozen Plasma
GOS	Glasgow Outcome Scale
GOS-E	Extended Glasgow Outcome Scale
GI	Gastrointestinal
HDU	High Dependency Unit
HES	Hydroxyethyl Starch

HFOV	High-Frequency Oscillatory Ventilation
HF	Heart Failure
HFNO	High-Flow Nasal Oxygen
HAS	Human Albumin Solution
HTX	Haemothorax
HVHF	High-Volume Haemofiltration
IABP	Intra-Aortic Balloon Pump
ICA	Internal Carotid Artery
ICH	Intracranial Haemorrhage
ICI	Invasive *Candida* Infection
ICP	Intracranial Pressure
ICU	Intensive Care Unit
IHD	Intermittent Haemodialysis
LOS	Length Of Stay
LV	Left Ventricular
LVAD	Left Ventricular Assist Device
LSD	Lower Severe Disability
MCA	Middle Cerebral Artery
MAKE	Major Adverse Kidney Events
MAP	Mean Arterial Pressure
MI	Myocardial Infarction
MgSO$_4$	Magnesium Sulphate
mRS	Modified Rankin Scale
MV	Mechanical Ventilation
NAC	N-Acetylcysteine
NA	Noradrenaline or norepinephrine
NG	Nasogastric
NIHSS	National Institutes of Health Stroke Scale
NIV	Non-Invasive Ventilation
NMB	Neuromuscular Blocker
NJ	Nasojejunal
OHCA	Out-of-Hospital Cardiac Arrest
PAC	Pulmonary Artery Catheter
PaCO$_2$	Partial Pressure of Carbon Dioxide
PaO$_2$	Partial Pressure of Oxygen
PCC	Prothrombin Complex Concentrate
PCV	Pressure-Controlled Ventilation

PE	Pulmonary Embolism
PEEP	Positive End-Expiratory Pressure
PEFR	Peak Expiratory Flow Rate
PN	Parenteral Nutrition
PPH	Post-Partum Haemorrhage
PTX	Pneumothorax
RBC	Red Blood Cell
RRT	Renal Replacement Therapy
ROSC	Return Of Spontaneous Circulation
SAH	Subarachnoid Haemorrhage
SaO$_2$	Arterial Oxygen Saturation
SCUF	Slow Continuous Ultrafiltration
SBP	Systolic Blood Pressure (when referring to blood pressure targets)
SBP	Spontaneous Bacterial Peritonitis
SDD	Selective Decontamination of the Digestive tract
SIRS	Systemic Inflammatory Response Syndrome
SLEDD	Slow Low-Efficiency Daily Dialysis
SOB	Shortness Of Breath
SOFA	Sequential Organ Failure Assessment
SNAP	Scottish and Newcastle Anti-emetic Pre-treatment for Paracetamol Poisoning
SpO$_2$	Peripheral Oxygen Saturation
SBT	Spontaneous Breathing Trial
SVHF	Standard-Volume Haemofiltration
TXA	Tranexamic Acid
TBI	Traumatic Brain Injury
UGIB	Upper Gastrointestinal Bleeding
USD	Upper Severe Disability
VAP	Ventilator-Associated Pneumonia
VA-ECMO	Veno-Arterial Extracorporeal Membrane Oxygenation
VL	Videolaryngoscope
VFDs	Ventilator-Free Days
VHA	Viscoelastic Haemostatic Assay
VKA-ICH	Vitamin K Antagonist–related Intracranial Haemorrhage

VENTILATORY STRATEGIES IN ARDS

Study Name	ARDSNet (2000)
Population	Patients with acute lung injury/ARDS
Intervention	Low tidal volume (V_T) of 4–6 ml/kg vs traditional V_T of 10–12 ml/kg
Primary Outcome/s	• **180-Day mortality**: Significantly lower with low V_T strategy • **Ventilator-free days (VFDs)**: Significantly more with low V_T strategy • **Breathing unaided by day 28**: Significantly higher with low V_T strategy
Secondary Outcome/s	• **Days without other organ failure**: Significantly higher with low V_T strategy
Viva Summary	In a study comparing low V_T ventilation (4–6 ml/kg) to traditional V_T (10–12 ml/kg) in patients with acute lung injury/ARDS, the low V_T strategy resulted in significantly lower 180-day mortality, more VFDs, a higher proportion breathing unaided by day 28, and more days without other organ failure.
Study Conclusion	'In patients with acute lung injury and ARDS, mechanical ventilation with a lower tidal volume than is traditionally used, results in decreased mortality and increases the number of days without ventilator use.'

ARDSNet (2000): The Acute Respiratory Distress Syndrome Network. Ventilation with lower tidal volumes as compared with traditional tidal volumes for acute lung injury and the acute respiratory distress syndrome. N Engl J Med. 2000;342(18):1301–1308.

DOI: 10.1201/9781003468738-1

Study Name	ALVEOLI (2004)
Population	Patients with acute lung injury and ARDS
Intervention	Higher PEEP vs lower PEEP (both strategies protocolised according to FiO_2, up to 24 cmH_2O)
Primary Outcome/s	• **Mortality before discharge home while breathing unaided**: No significant difference
Secondary Outcome/s	• **Breathing without assistance at day 28, VFDs, Days not in ICU, Barotrauma, Days without organ failure**: No significant difference
Viva Summary	In a study involving patients with acute lung injury and ARDS, the comparison of higher PEEP and lower PEEP interventions, both adjusted according to FiO_2, with a maximum of 24 cmH_2O, showed no significant difference in primary outcome, which was mortality before discharge home while breathing unaided. Additionally, there were no significant differences in various secondary outcomes, including the ability to breathe without assistance at day 28, VFDs, days outside the ICU, barotrauma, and days without organ failure.
Study Conclusion	'These results suggest that in patients with acute lung injury and ARDS who receive mechanical ventilation with a tidal-volume goal of 6 ml per kilogram of predicted body weight and an end-inspiratory plateau-pressure limit of 30 cm of water, clinical outcomes are similar whether lower or higher PEEP levels are used.'

ALVEOLI (2004): The National Heart, Lung, and Blood Institute ARDS Clinical Trials Network. Higher versus lower positive end-expiratory pressures in patients with the acute respiratory distress syndrome. N Engl J Med. 2004;351(4):327–336.

Study Name	OSCILLATE (2013)
Population	Patients with new-onset moderate-to-severe ARDS
Intervention	High-frequency oscillatory ventilation (HFOV) vs conventional PCV
Primary Outcome/s	• **In-hospital mortality**: Significantly higher in HFOV group • Trial was terminated early
Secondary Outcome/s	• **Refractory hypoxaemia**: Lower in HFOV group • **Use of NMBs, midazolam, and vasoactive drugs**: Higher in HFOV group
Viva Summary	In a study comparing HFOV to conventional PCV in patients with new-onset moderate-to-severe ARDS, the HFOV group had significantly higher in-hospital mortality despite lower rates of refractory hypoxaemia, leading to the early termination of the trial. The HFOV group also required higher use of neuromuscular blockers, midazolam, and vasoactive drugs compared to the conventional PCV group.
Study Conclusion	'In adults with moderate-to-severe ARDS, early application of HFOV, as compared with a ventilation strategy of low tidal volume and high positive end-expiratory pressure, does not reduce, and may increase, in-hospital mortality.'

OSCILLATE (2013): Ferguson ND, Cook DJ, Guyatt GH, et al. High-frequency oscillation in early acute respiratory distress syndrome. N Engl J Med. 2013;368(9):795–805.

Study Name	OSCAR (2013)
Population	Patients with ARDS
Intervention	HFOV vs local practice
Primary Outcome/s	• **30-Day mortality**: No significant difference
Secondary Outcome/s	• **Oxygenation, NMBs duration**: Significantly higher in the HFOV group • **VFDs, ICU/hospital LOS, Antimicrobial/inotrope/ vasopressor/sedation duration**: No significant difference
Viva Summary	In a study comparing HFOV to standard local practice in patients with ARDS, there was no significant difference in 30-day mortality between the two groups. However, the HFOV group showed significantly higher oxygenation and a longer duration of neuromuscular blockade, while other outcomes such as VFDs and ICU/hospital LOS did not differ significantly between the groups.
Study Conclusion	'The use of HFOV had no significant effect on 30-day mortality in patients undergoing mechanical ventilation for ARDS.'

OSCAR (2013): Young D, Lamb SW, Shah S, et al. High-frequency oscillation for acute respiratory distress syndrome. N Engl J Med. 2013;368(9):806–813.

Study Name	Kacmarek et al. (2016)
Population	Patients with established moderate/severe ARDS
Intervention	Open lung approach (moderate-to-high levels of PEEP) vs ARDS network protocol
Primary Outcome/s	• **60-Day mortality**: No significant difference
Secondary Outcome/s	• **ICU mortality, VFDs, Major adverse events**: No significant difference • Post-hoc analysis: The open lung group showed a significant improvement in PaO_2/FiO_2 ratio at 24 hours, and at day 3, lower plateau pressure, PEEP, driving pressure, and FiO_2 requirement
Viva Summary	In a study comparing an open lung approach (moderate-to-high levels of PEEP) to the ARDS network protocol in patients with established moderate/severe ARDS, there was no significant difference in 60-day mortality, ICU mortality, VFDs, or major adverse events. However, post-hoc analysis revealed that the open lung group exhibited a significant improvement in PaO_2/FiO_2 ratio at 24 hours and lower plateau pressure, PEEP, driving pressure, and FiO_2 requirement by day 3.
Study Conclusion	'In patients with established acute respiratory distress syndrome, open lung approach improved oxygenation and driving pressure, without detrimental effects on mortality, ventilator-free days, or barotrauma. This pilot study supports the need for a large, multicenter trial using recruitment maneuvers and a decremental positive end-expiratory pressure trial in persistent acute respiratory distress syndrome.'

Kacmarek RM, Villar J, Sulemanji D, Montiel R, et al.; Open Lung Approach Network. Open lung approach for the acute respiratory distress syndrome: a pilot, randomized controlled trial. Crit Care Med. 2016 Jan;44(1):32–42.

PRONING IN ARDS

Study Name	PROSEVA (2013)
Population	Patients with severe ARDS
Intervention	Prone positioning for ≥16 hours for 28 days or until improvement vs supine
Primary Outcome/s	• **28-Day all-cause mortality**: Significantly lower in prone group
Secondary Outcome/s	• **Unadjusted 90-day mortality**: Significantly lower in prone group • **Adverse events**: No significant difference
Viva Summary	In a study comparing prone positioning for at least 16 hours a day for 28 days (or until improvement) versus supine positioning in patients with severe ARDS, the prone group showed significantly lower 28-day and 90-day mortality rates. There was no significant difference in adverse events between the two groups.
Study Conclusion	'In patients with severe ARDS, early application of prolonged prone-positioning sessions significantly decreased 28-day and 90-day mortality.'

PROSEVA (2013): Guérin C, Reignier J, Richard JC, et al. Prone positioning in severe acute respiratory distress syndrome. N Engl J Med. 2013;368(23): 2159–2168.

NEUROMUSCULAR BLOCKADE IN ARDS

Study Name	ACURASYS (2010)
Population	Patients with moderate-severe ARDS
Intervention	Cisatracurium for 48 hours vs placebo
Primary Outcome/s	• **Adjusted 90-day mortality**: Significantly lower with cisatracurium • **Actual 90-day mortality**: No significant difference
Secondary Outcome/s	• **Barotrauma, PTX**: Significantly lower with cisatracurium • **Days with non-respiratory organ failure**: Significantly higher with cisatracurium • **ICU-acquired paresis**: No significant difference
Viva Summary	In a study involving patients with moderate-severe ARDS, the intervention of using cisatracurium for 48 hours resulted in a significantly lower adjusted 90-day mortality rate compared to placebo. However, there was no significant difference in actual 90-day mortality. Cisatracurium also led to significantly lower rates of barotrauma and PTX but increased the number of days with non-respiratory organ failure, while there was no significant difference in ICU-acquired paresis.
Study Conclusion	'In patients with severe ARDS, early administration of a neuromuscular blocking agent improved the adjusted 90-day survival and increased the time off the ventilator without increasing muscle weakness.'

ACURASYS (2010): Papazian L, Forel J-M, Gacouin A, et al. Neuromuscular blockers in early acute respiratory distress syndrome. N Engl J Med. 2010;363(12):1107–1116.

Study Name	ROSE (2019)
Population	Patients with moderate-to-severe ARDS
Intervention	Cisatracurium infusion for 48 hours vs usual care
Primary Outcome/s	• **90-Day mortality**: No significant difference • The study was stopped early due to futility
Secondary Outcome/s	• Occurrence of serious cardiovascular events was higher in the cisatracurium group • No significant differences were seen in other secondary outcomes, including 28-day mortality, days free of mechanical ventilation, ICU-free days, hospital-free days, ICU-acquired weakness, VFDs, and long-term quality of life
Viva Summary	In a study involving patients with moderate-to-severe ARDS, a 48-hour infusion of cisatracurium showed no significant difference in 90-day mortality compared to usual care, leading to the study being prematurely stopped due to futility. However, the cisatracurium group experienced a higher occurrence of serious cardiovascular events. Other secondary outcomes, including 28-day mortality, days free from mechanical ventilation, ICU-free days, hospital-free days, ICU-acquired weakness, and long-term quality of life, showed no significant differences.
Study Conclusion	'Among patients with moderate-to-severe ARDS who were treated with a strategy involving a high PEEP, there was no significant difference in mortality at 90 days between patients who received an early and continuous cisatracurium infusion and those who were treated with a usual-care approach with lighter sedation targets.'

ROSE (2019): The National Heart, Lung, and Blood Institute PETAL Clinical Trials Network. Early neuromuscular blockade in the acute respiratory distress syndrome. N Engl J Med. 2019;380(21):1997–2008.

CORTICOSTEROIDS IN ARDS

Study Name	Meduri et al. (2007)
Population	Patients with early severe ARDS
Intervention	Methylprednisolone infusion (1 mg/kg/day) vs placebo
Primary Outcome/s	• **1-Point reduction in Lung Injury Score or successful extubation by day 7**: Significantly higher with methylprednisolone
Secondary Outcome/s	• **Duration of mechanical ventilation, ICU LOS, ICU mortality, Infections**: Significantly lower with methylprednisolone
Viva Summary	In a study involving patients with early severe ARDS, the intervention of methylprednisolone infusion (1 mg/kg/day) was compared to a placebo. The primary outcome, which was a 1-point reduction in Lung Injury Score or successful extubation by day 7, was significantly better in the methylprednisolone group. Additionally, secondary outcomes, including the duration of mechanical ventilation, ICU LOS, ICU mortality, and infections, were significantly lower in the methylprednisolone group.
Study Conclusion	'Methylprednisolone-induced down-regulation of systemic inflammation was associated with significant improvement in pulmonary and extrapulmonary organ dysfunction and reduction in duration of mechanical ventilation and ICU length of stay.'

Meduri GU, Golden E, Freire AX, et al. Methylprednisolone infusion in early severe ARDS: results of a randomized controlled trial. Chest. 2007;131(4): 954–963.

Study Name	DEXA-ARDS (2020)
Population	Patients with moderate-severe ARDS
Intervention	IV dexamethasone (20 mg daily for 5 days, followed by 10 mg daily up to day 10 or until extubation) vs conventional treatment
Primary Outcome/s	• **VFDs**: Significantly higher with dexamethasone
Secondary Outcome/s	• **60-Day mortality, ICU mortality**: Significantly lower with dexamethasone
Viva Summary	In a study involving patients with moderate-severe ARDS, the use of IV dexamethasone (20 mg daily for 5 days, followed by 10 mg daily up to day 10 or until extubation) led to significantly more VFDs and significantly lower 60-day and ICU mortality compared to conventional treatment.
Study Conclusion	'Early administration of dexamethasone could reduce duration of mechanical ventilation and overall mortality in patients with established moderate-to-severe ARDS.'

DEXA-ARDS (2020): Villar J, Ferrando C, Martínez C, et al. Dexamethasone treatment for the acute respiratory distress syndrome: a multicentre, randomised controlled trial. Lancet Respir Med. 2020;8(3):267–276.

EXTRACORPOREAL MEMBRANE OXYGENATION (ECMO) IN ARDS

Study Name	CESAR (2009)
Population	Adults with severe, potentially reversible respiratory failure
Intervention	Transfer to specialist centre and consideration for ECMO vs conventional PCV
Primary Outcome/s	• **Survival without severe disability at 6 months**: Significantly higher in ECMO group
Secondary Outcome/s	• **ICU/Hospital LOS**: Higher in the ECMO group
Viva Summary	In a study involving adults with severe, potentially reversible respiratory failure, those transferred to a specialist centre and considered for ECMO showed significantly higher survival without severe disability at 6 months compared to those receiving conventional PCV. However, the ECMO group had a longer ICU/hospital LOS as a secondary outcome.
Study Conclusion	'We recommend transferring of adult patients with severe but potentially reversible respiratory failure, whose Murray score exceeds 3.0 or who have a pH of less than 7.20 on optimum conventional management, to a centre with an ECMO-based management protocol to significantly improve survival without severe disability. This strategy is also likely to be cost effective in settings with similar services to those in the UK.'

CESAR (2009): Peek GJ, Mugford M, Tiruvoipati R, et al. Efficacy and economic assessment of conventional ventilatory support versus extracorporeal membrane oxygenation for severe adult respiratory failure (CESAR): a multicentre randomised controlled trial. Lancet. 2009;374(9698):1351–1363.

Study Name	EOLIA (2018)
Population	Adults with severe ARDS
Intervention	VV-ECMO vs conventional mechanical ventilation
Primary Outcome/s	• **60-Day mortality**: No significant difference
Secondary Outcome/s	• **60-Day treatment failure, RRT at day 60**: Lower relative risk in VV-ECMO group • **Proning**: ECMO patients underwent less proning • Cross-over to ECMO occurred in 28% of control patients
Viva Summary	In a study comparing VV-ECMO with conventional mechanical ventilation for adults with severe ARDS, there was no significant difference in 60-day mortality. However, the VV-ECMO group had a lower relative risk of 60-day treatment failure and the need for RRT, and they also required less proning compared to the conventional ventilation group.
Study Conclusion	'Among patients with very severe ARDS, 60-day mortality was not significantly lower with ECMO than with a strategy of conventional mechanical ventilation that included ECMO as rescue therapy.'

EOLIA (2018): Combes A, Hajage D, Capellier G, et al. Extracorporeal membrane oxygenation for severe acute respiratory distress syndrome. N Engl J Med. 2018;378(21):1965–1975.

EXTRACORPOREAL CARBON DIOXIDE REMOVAL (ECCO$_2$R)

Study Name	SUPERNOVA (2019)
Population	Patients with ARDS
Evaluation	Three ECCO$_2$R (extracorporeal carbon dioxide removal) systems: Hemolung, Novalung, Cardiohelp evaluated for ability to facilitate ultra-protective ventilation
Primary Outcome/s	Number of patients achieving ultra-protective ventilation (V_T 4 ml/kg with PaCO$_2$ ≤20% of baseline and pH >7.30): • Achieved in 78% of patients at 8 hours • Achieved in 82% of patients at 24 hours
Secondary Outcome/s	• 73% of patients were alive at day 28 • 62% of patients were alive at hospital discharge • Adverse events occurred in 39% of cases, including membrane lung clot (14%), thrombocytopaenia (13%), haemolysis (12%), significant bleeding (6%), pump malfunction (3%), line displacement (2%), and infection (2%) • Six severe adverse events were reported, with two attributed to ECCO$_2$R (Massive ICH and PTX)
Viva Summary	In patients with ARDS, three CCO$_2$R systems (Hemolung, Novalung, Cardiohelp) achieved ultra-protective ventilation in 78% of patients at 8 hours and 82% at 24 hours. Survival rates were reported as 73% at day 28, with 62% of patients surviving to hospital discharge. Adverse events were documented in 39% of the patients.
Study Conclusion	'Use of ECCO$_2$R to facilitate ultra-protective ventilation was feasible. A randomized clinical trial is required to assess the overall benefits and harms.'

SUPERNOVA (2019): Combes A, Fanelli V, Pham T, et al. Feasibility and safety of extracorporeal CO$_2$ removal to enhance protective ventilation in acute respiratory distress syndrome: the SUPERNOVA study. Intensive Care Med. 2019;45(5):592–600.

Study Name	REST (2021)
Population	Acute hypoxaemic respiratory failure
Intervention	$ECCO_2R$ (using dual-lumen catheter and heparinised) vs guideline-based mechanical ventilation
Primary Outcome/s	• **90-Day all-cause mortality**: No significant difference
Secondary Outcome/s	• **28-Day mortality, ICU/Hospital LOS**: No significant difference • **V_T on Days 2–3, VFDs**: Significantly lower in $ECCO_2R$ group
Viva Summary	In a study comparing $ECCO_2R$ to guideline-based mechanical ventilation for acute hypoxaemic respiratory failure, there was no significant difference in 90-day all-cause mortality, 28-day mortality, or ICU/hospital LOS. However, the $ECCO_2R$ group had significantly lower V_T on days 2–3 and fewer VFDs.
Study Conclusion	'Among patients with acute hypoxemic respiratory failure, the use of extracorporeal carbon dioxide removal to facilitate lower tidal volume mechanical ventilation, compared with conventional low tidal volume mechanical ventilation, did not significantly reduce 90-day mortality. However, due to early termination, the study may have been underpowered to detect a clinically important difference.'

REST (2021): McNamee JJ, Gillies MA, Barrett NA, et al. Effect of lower tidal volume ventilation facilitated by extracorporeal carbon dioxide removal vs standard care ventilation on 90-day mortality in patients with acute hypoxemic respiratory failure: the REST randomized clinical trial. JAMA. 2021;326(11):1013–1023.

OXYGENATION TARGETS

Study Name	ICU-ROX (2019)
Population	Mechanically ventilated ICU patients
Intervention	Conservative oxygen therapy (target S_aO_2 90–97%) vs usual therapy (no upper limit)
Primary Outcome/s	• **VFDs**: No significant difference
Secondary Outcome/s	• **180-Day mortality, Cognitive function, Quality of life, Employment status**: No significant difference • **Subgroup analysis of 180-day mortality**: – **In ischaemic hypoxic encephalopathy**: Mortality significantly lower in the conservative oxygen group – **In sepsis and other brain pathology**: Mortality significantly higher in the conservative oxygen group
Viva Summary	In a study comparing conservative oxygen therapy (targeting S_aO_2 90–97%) to usual therapy (no upper limit) among mechanically ventilated ICU patients, there were no significant differences observed in VFDs or in secondary outcomes such as cognitive function, quality of life, and employment status. Subgroup analysis revealed that in cases of ischaemic hypoxic encephalopathy, mortality was significantly lower with conservative oxygen therapy, while in sepsis and other brain pathologies, mortality was significantly higher.
Study Conclusion	'In adults undergoing mechanical ventilation in the ICU, the use of conservative oxygen therapy, as compared with usual oxygen therapy, did not significantly affect the number of ventilator-free days.'

ICU-ROX (2019): The ICU-ROX Investigators and the Australian and New Zealand Intensive Care Society Clinical Trials Group. Conservative oxygen therapy during mechanical ventilation in the ICU. N Engl J Med. 2020; 382(11):989–998.

Study Name	HOT-ICU (2021)
Population	ICU patients receiving oxygen ≥10 l/min or FiO$_2$ ≥0.5 in a closed system
Intervention	Target oxygenation levels: conservative (8 kPa) vs liberal (12 kPa)
Primary Outcome/s	• **90-Day mortality**: No significant difference
Secondary Outcome/s	• **Days alive without life support, Days alive after hospital discharge, Serious adverse events**: No significant difference
Viva Summary	In a study comparing conservative (8 kPa) and liberal (12 kPa) oxygenation levels for ICU patients receiving oxygen in a closed system, there was no significant difference in 90-day mortality rates. Additionally, no significant differences were observed in days alive without life support, days alive after hospital discharge, or serious adverse events.
Study Conclusion	'Among adult patients with acute hypoxemic respiratory failure in the ICU, a lower oxygenation target did not result in lower mortality than a higher target at 90 days.'

HOT-ICU (2021): Schjørring OL, Klitgaard TL, Perner A, et al. Lower or higher oxygenation targets for acute hypoxemic respiratory failure. N Engl J Med. 2021;384(14):1301–1311.

Study Name	PILOT (2022)
Population	Patients receiving invasive mechanical ventilation
Intervention	Lower oxygen target (S_pO_2 90%) and intermediate oxygen target (S_pO_2 94%) vs higher oxygen target (S_pO_2 98%)
Primary Outcome/s	• **Number of days alive and ventilator-free at 28 days**: No significant difference
Secondary Outcome/s	• No significant difference in secondary outcomes or numerous prespecified exploratory outcomes, including in-hospital mortality at 28 days
Viva Summary	In a study comparing different oxygen targets for patients on invasive mechanical ventilation, lower and intermediate oxygen levels (S_pO_2 90% and 94%) were found to have no significant difference in the number of days alive and ventilator-free at 28 days compared to higher oxygen levels (S_pO_2 98%). Additionally, there were no significant differences in secondary or exploratory outcomes, including in-hospital mortality at 28 days.
Study Conclusion	'Among critically ill adults receiving invasive mechanical ventilation, the number of ventilator-free days did not differ among groups in which a lower, intermediate, or higher SpO_2 target was used.'

PILOT (2022): Semler MW, Casey JD, Lloyd BD, Hastings PG et al.; PILOT Investigators and the Pragmatic Critical Care Research Group. Oxygen saturation targets for critically ill adults receiving mechanical ventilation. N Engl J Med. 2022 Nov 10;387(19):1759–1769.

Study Name	BOX (Oxygen) (2022)
Population	Comatose patients following cardiac arrest
Intervention	Restrictive oxygenation (P_aO_2 9–10 kPa) vs liberal oxygenation (P_aO_2 13–14 kPa)
Primary Outcome/s	• **Composite of death or discharge from hospital with severe disability or coma (Cerebral Performance Category of 3 or 4) within 90 days of randomisation**: No significant difference
Secondary Outcome/s	• **Death within 90 days, Acute kidney injury with RRT, CPC at 90 days, Montreal Cognitive Assessment score at 90 days, Neuron-specific enolase at 48 hours**: No significant difference
Viva Summary	In a study involving comatose patients after cardiac arrest, a comparison was made between restrictive oxygenation (P_aO_2 9–10 kPa) and liberal oxygenation (P_aO_2 13–14 kPa). The primary outcome, which was a composite of death or discharge from the hospital with severe disability or coma within 90 days, showed no significant difference between the two groups. Additionally, secondary outcomes such as death within 90 days, acute kidney injury with RRT, CPC at 90 days, Montreal Cognitive Assessment score at 90 days, and neuron-specific enolase at 48 hours also did not show any significant differences.
Study Conclusion	'Targeting of a restrictive or liberal oxygenation strategy in comatose patients after resuscitation for cardiac arrest resulted in a similar incidence of death or severe disability or coma.'

BOX (2022): Schmidt H, Kjaergaard J, Hassager C, Mølstrøm S, et al. Oxygen targets in comatose survivors of cardiac arrest. N Engl J Med. 2022 Oct 20;387(16):1467–1476.

RESPIRATORY WEANING

Study Name	TracMan (2013)
Population	Mechanically ventilated adults at high risk of prolonged ventilation
Intervention	Tracheostomy insertion: early ≤4 days vs late ≥10 days (if still required)
Primary Outcome/s	• **30-Day all-cause mortality**: No significant difference
Secondary Outcome/s	• **Survival, Duration of mechanical ventilation, ICU LOS, Use of antibiotics**: No significant difference • **Days of sedation in survivors at 30 days**: Significantly less in the early tracheostomy group
Viva Summary	In a study involving adults who were mechanically ventilated and at high risk of requiring prolonged ventilation, the timing of tracheostomy insertion—either early (within 4 days) or late (after 10 days, if still required)—was compared. The primary outcome, 30-day all-cause mortality, showed no significant difference between the two groups. Additionally, there were no significant differences in secondary outcomes, including survival, duration of mechanical ventilation, ICU LOS, and antibiotic use. However, survivors in the early tracheostomy group experienced significantly fewer sedation days at 30 days compared to those in the late group.
Study Conclusion	'For patients breathing with the aid of mechanical ventilation treated in adult critical care units in the United Kingdom, tracheostomy within 4 days of critical care admission was not associated with an improvement in 30-day mortality or other important secondary outcomes. The ability of clinicians to predict which patients required extended ventilatory support was limited.'

TracMan (2013): Young D, Harrison DA, Cuthbertson BH, et al. Effect of early vs late tracheostomy placement on survival in patients receiving mechanical ventilation. JAMA. 2013;309(20):2121–2129.

Study Name	*Hernández et al. (2016)*
Population	Extubated patients at low risk for reintubation
Intervention	HFNO vs conventional oxygen therapy for 24 hours after extubation
Primary Outcome/s	• **Reintubation within 72 hours**: Significantly lower in the HFNO group
Secondary Outcome/s	• **Post-extubation respiratory failure**: Significantly lower in the HFNO group • **Time to reintubation**: No significant difference
Viva Summary	In a study comparing HFNO to conventional oxygen therapy for 24 hours after extubation in low-risk patients, the HFNO group had significantly fewer cases of reintubation within 72 hours and lower rates of post-extubation respiratory failure. However, there was no significant difference in the time to reintubation between the two groups.
Study Conclusion	'Among extubated patients at low risk for reintubation, the use of high-flow nasal cannula oxygen compared with conventional oxygen therapy reduced the risk of reintubation within 72 hours.'

Hernández G, Vaquero C, González P, Subira C, et al. Effect of postextubation high-flow nasal cannula vs conventional oxygen therapy on reintubation in low-risk patients: a randomized clinical trial. JAMA. 2016 Apr 5;315(13): 1354–1361.

Study Name	Subirà et al. (2019)
Population	Adults ready for weaning after ≥24 hours of mechanical ventilation
Intervention	30-Min 8 cmH_2O pressure support spontaneous breathing trial (SBT) vs 2-hour T-piece SBT
Primary Outcome/s	• **Successful extubation (remaining free of mechanical ventilation 72 hours after first SBT)**: Significantly higher in pressure support group
Secondary Outcome/s	• **Hospital/90-Day mortality**: Significantly lower in the pressure support group • **Reintubation, ICU/Hospital LOS**: No significant difference
Viva Summary	In a study comparing two weaning methods for adults on mechanical ventilation, a 30-minute 8 cmH_2O pressure support SBT resulted in significantly higher successful extubation rates after 72 hours compared to a 2-hour T-piece SBT. Additionally, the pressure support group had significantly lower hospital/90-day mortality rates, with no significant differences in reintubation or ICU/hospital LOS observed between the two groups.
Study Conclusion	'Among patients receiving mechanical ventilation, a spontaneous breathing trial consisting of 30 minutes of pressure support ventilation, compared with 2 hours of T-piece ventilation, led to significantly higher rates of successful extubation. These findings support the use of a shorter, less demanding ventilation strategy for spontaneous breathing trials.'

Subirà C, Hernández G, Vásquez A, et al. Effect of pressure support vs T-piece ventilation strategies during spontaneous breathing trials on successful extubation among patients receiving mechanical ventilation: a randomized clinical trial. JAMA. 2019;321(22):2175–2182.

ASTHMA

Study Name	3Mg (2013)
Population	Patients with severe acute asthma (excluding life-threatening/near-fatal asthma)
Intervention	IV $MgSO_4$ vs nebulised $MgSO_4$ vs placebo
Primary Outcome/s	• **Hospital admission rate, Breathlessness**: No significant difference
Secondary Outcome/s	• **Mortality, Respiratory Support, Hospital LOS, HDU/ICU Admission, Change in PEFR/Physiological Variables**: No significant difference
Viva Summary	In a study involving patients with severe acute asthma, the use of IV $MgSO_4$ compared to nebulised $MgSO_4$ or a placebo did not show any significant differences in outcomes. These outcomes included hospital admission rates, breathlessness, mortality, respiratory support, hospital length of stay, HDU/ICU admission, and changes in PEFR and physiological variables.
Study Conclusion	'Our findings suggest nebulised $MgSO_4$ has no role in the management of severe acute asthma in adults and at best suggest only a limited role for intravenous $MgSO_4$ in this setting.'

3Mg (2013): Goodacre S, Cohen J, Bradburn M, et al. Intravenous or nebulised magnesium sulphate versus standard therapy for severe acute asthma (3Mg trial): a double-blind, randomised controlled trial. Lancet Respir Med. 2013;1(4):293–300.

CYSTIC FIBROSIS

Study Name	Middleton et al. (2019)
Population	Patients with cystic fibrosis, heterozygous Phe508del CFTR mutation, age ≥12 years
Intervention	Elexacaftor–tezacaftor–ivacaftor treatment vs placebo
Primary Outcome/s	• **Absolute change in % predicted FEV$_1$ at 4 weeks**: Significantly higher in treatment group
Secondary Outcome/s	• **Exacerbations, Sweat chloride concentration**: Significantly lower in treatment group • **Quality of life**: Significantly higher in treatment group
Viva Summary	In a study involving patients with cystic fibrosis aged ≥12 years and heterozygous for the Phe508del CFTR mutation, elexacaftor–tezacaftor–ivacaftor treatment was compared to a placebo. The primary outcome, which was the absolute change in % predicted FEV$_1$ after 4 weeks, showed a significant improvement in the treatment group. Additionally, secondary outcomes such as exacerbations, sweat chloride concentration, and quality of life were also significantly better in the treatment group.
Study Conclusion	'Elexacaftor–tezacaftor–ivacaftor was efficacious in patients with cystic fibrosis with Phe508del–minimal function genotypes, in whom previous CFTR modulator regimens were ineffective.'

Middleton PG, Mall MA, Dřevínek P, et al. Elexacaftor–tezacaftor–ivacaftor for cystic fibrosis with a single Phe508del allele. N Engl J Med. 2019;381(19): 1809–1819.

ACUTE HYPOXAEMIC RESPIRATORY FAILURE

Study Name	Delclaux et al. (2000)
Population	Patients with acute hypoxaemic, non-hypercapnic, respiratory insufficiency
Intervention	Addition of CPAP vs conventional oxygen therapy
Primary Outcome/s	• **Rate of tracheal intubation**: No significant difference
Secondary Outcome/s	• **ICU LOS, Hospital mortality**: No significant difference • **Respiratory indices (Subjective response to treatment, P/F ratio)**: Improved at 1 hour in CPAP group, then no difference • **Adverse events**: Significantly higher in CPAP group
Viva Summary	In a study involving patients with acute hypoxemic, non-hypercapnic respiratory insufficiency, the addition of CPAP compared to conventional oxygen therapy did not result in a significant difference in the rate of tracheal intubation, ICU LOS, or hospital mortality. While respiratory indices initially improved in the CPAP group at 1 hour, there was no significant difference after that time. The CPAP group also experienced significantly more adverse events compared to the conventional oxygen therapy group.
Study Conclusion	'In this study, despite early physiologic improvement, CPAP neither reduced the need for intubation nor improved outcomes in patients with acute hypoxemic, non-hypercapnic respiratory insufficiency primarily due to acute lung injury.'

Delclaux C, L'Her E, Alberti C, et al. Treatment of acute hypoxemic nonhyper-capnic respiratory insufficiency with continuous positive airway pressure delivered by a face mask: a randomized controlled trial. JAMA. 2000;284(18): 2352–2360.

Study Name	FLORALI (2015)
Population	Patients with acute hypoxaemic respiratory failure
Intervention	HFNO vs NIV vs facemask oxygen
Primary Outcome/s	• **Rate of tracheal intubation**: No significant difference
Secondary Outcome/s	• **90-Day mortality, Discomfort at 1 hour**: Significantly lower with HFNO • **ICU LOS, Complications**: No significant difference
Viva Summary	In a study comparing treatments for patients with acute hypoxaemic respiratory failure, the primary outcome, the rate of tracheal intubation, showed no significant difference between HFNO, NIV, and facemask oxygen. However, secondary outcomes revealed that HFNO led to significantly lower 90-day mortality and less discomfort at 1 hour compared to the other interventions, while there were no significant differences in ICU LOS or rate of complications.
Study Conclusion	'In patients with nonhypercapnic acute hypoxemic respiratory failure, treatment with high-flow oxygen, standard oxygen, or noninvasive ventilation did not result in significantly different intubation rates. There was a significant difference in favor of high-flow oxygen in 90-day mortality.'

FLORALI (2015): Frat JP, Whille AW, Mercat A, et al. High-flow oxygen through nasal cannula in acute hypoxemic respiratory failure. N Engl J Med. 2015;372(23):2185–2196.

COMMUNITY-ACQUIRED PNEUMONIA

Study Name	CAPE COD (2023)
Population	ICU patients with severe community-acquired pneumonia
Intervention	Hydrocortisone 200 mg/day for 4 days vs placebo
Primary Outcome/s	• **28-Day mortality**: Significantly reduced in the hydrocortisone group
Secondary Outcome/s	• **90-Day mortality**: Reduced in the hydrocortisone group • **Endotracheal intubation and vasopressor initiation**: Reduced in selected subgroups within the hydrocortisone group • **Daily dose of insulin**: Higher in the hydrocortisone group • **Hospital-acquired infection, GI bleeding**: No significant difference
Viva Summary	In a study on ICU patients with severe community-acquired pneumonia, the administration of hydrocortisone 200 mg/day for 4 days significantly reduced 28-day mortality compared to a placebo. Additionally, the hydrocortisone group had better 90-day survival and decreased rates of endotracheal intubation and vasopressor initiation in selected subgroups. The hydrocortisone group did need a higher daily dose of insulin, but other complications such as hospital-acquired infection and GI bleeding were not significantly different.
Study Conclusion	'Among patients with severe community-acquired pneumonia being treated in the ICU, those who received hydrocortisone had a lower risk of death by day 28 than those who received placebo.'

CAPE COD (2023): Dequin PF, Meziani F, Quenot JP, Kamel T, et al. Hydrocortisone in severe community-acquired pneumonia. N Engl J Med. 2023 May 25;388(21):1931–1941.

COPD

Study Name	DIABOLO (2016)
Population	Critically ill patients with COPD and metabolic alkalosis
Intervention	Acetazolamide for up to 28 days vs placebo
Primary Outcome/s	• **Duration of invasive ventilation:** No significant difference
Secondary Outcome/s	• **Serum bicarbonate, Days with metabolic alkalosis:** Significantly lower in acetazolamide group • **Duration of weaning off invasive ventilation, Number of SBTs, Use of tracheostomy or NIV after extubation, VAP episodes, ICU LOS, ICU mortality:** No significant difference
Viva Summary	A study compared critically ill COPD patients with metabolic alkalosis who were treated with acetazolamide for up to 28 days against those given a placebo. There was no significant difference in the duration of invasive ventilation between the groups. However, the acetazolamide group exhibited lower serum bicarbonate levels and fewer days with metabolic alkalosis as secondary outcomes. Weaning duration and other ICU outcomes showed no significant differences between the groups.
Study Conclusion	'Among patients with COPD receiving invasive mechanical ventilation, the use of acetazolamide, compared with placebo, did not result in a statistically significant reduction in the duration of invasive mechanical ventilation. However, the magnitude of the difference was clinically important, and it is possible that the study was underpowered to establish statistical significance.'

DIABOLO (2016): Faisy C, Meziani F, Planquette B, et al. Effect of acetazolamide vs placebo on duration of invasive mechanical ventilation among patients with chronic obstructive pulmonary disease: a randomized clinical trial. JAMA. 2016;315(5):480–488.

COVID-19

Study Name	REMAP-CAP (2020) Corticosteroid
Population	Severe COVID-19
Intervention	Hydrocortisone with two arms—fixed dose (50 mg every 6 hours for 7 days) and shock-dependent (50 mg every 6 hours while in clinically evident shock) vs standard care
Primary Outcome/s	• **Respiratory/Cardiovascular support-free days up to day 21**: No significant difference • The probability that hydrocortisone was beneficial was 93% for the fixed-dose group and 80% for the shock-dependent group, but neither met the criteria for statistical superiority • Trial stopped early
Secondary Outcome/s	• Various secondary outcomes were assessed, including in-hospital mortality, time to death and ICU/hospital LOS. None of these secondary outcomes showed a clear benefit of hydrocortisone over no hydrocortisone
Viva Summary	In a study comparing two methods of administering hydrocortisone to severe COVID-19 patients, neither the fixed-dose nor the shock-dependent approach showed a significant advantage in terms of respiratory and cardiovascular support-free days up to day 21. The trial was stopped prematurely, and various secondary outcomes, such as in-hospital mortality and ICU/hospital LOS, did not demonstrate a clear benefit of hydrocortisone treatment over standard care.
Study Conclusion	'Among patients with severe COVID-19, treatment with a 7-day fixed-dose course of hydrocortisone or shock-dependent dosing of hydrocortisone, compared with no hydrocortisone, resulted in 93% and 80% probabilities of superiority with regard to the odds of improvement in organ support–free days within 21 days. However, the trial was stopped early and no treatment strategy met prespecified criteria for statistical superiority, precluding definitive conclusions.'

REMAP-CAP (2020) Corticosteroid: The Writing Committee for the REMAP-CAP Investigators. Effect of hydrocortisone on mortality and organ support in patients with severe COVID-19: the REMAP-CAP COVID-19 corticosteroid domain randomized clinical trial. JAMA. 2020;324(13):1317–1329.

Study Name	RECOVERY (2021) Dexamethasone
Population	Hospitalised patients with SARS-CoV-2 infection
Intervention	Dexamethasone (6 mg daily for 10 days) vs usual care
Primary Outcome/s	• **28-Day mortality**: Significantly lower in dexamethasone group
Secondary Outcome/s	28-Day mortality in subgroups: • **Patients receiving mechanical ventilation or supplemental oxygen**: Significantly lower in dexamethasone group • **Symptoms >7 days and were more likely to be receiving invasive mechanical ventilation**: Significantly lower in dexamethasone group • **Patients not receiving respiratory support**: No significant difference Other secondary outcomes: • **Composite of invasive mechanical ventilation and death, Use of mechanical ventilation, Hospital LOS**: Significantly lower in dexamethasone group
Viva Summary	In a study comparing dexamethasone (6 mg daily for 10 days) to usual care in hospitalised SARS-CoV-2 patients, the dexamethasone group had significantly lower 28-day mortality rates. This effect was more pronounced in patients on mechanical ventilation or supplemental oxygen and those with symptoms lasting over 7 days requiring invasive mechanical ventilation. Additionally, dexamethasone reduced the need for mechanical ventilation, shortened hospital LOS, and lowered the composite risk of invasive mechanical ventilation and death. There was no significant difference in outcome in patients not requiring respiratory support.
Study Conclusion	'In patients hospitalized with Covid-19, the use of dexamethasone resulted in lower 28-day mortality among those who were receiving either invasive mechanical ventilation or oxygen alone at randomization but not among those receiving no respiratory support.'

RECOVERY (2021) Dexamethasone: The RECOVERY Collaborative Group, Dexamethasone in hospitalized patients with Covid-19. N Engl J Med. 2021;384(8):693–704.

Study Name	REMAP-CAP (2021) IL-6
Population	Critically ill COVID-19 patients receiving organ support on ICU
Intervention	Tocilizumab vs sarilumab vs standard care
Primary Outcome/s	• **Organ support-free days up to day 21**: Significantly increased in both Tocilizumab and Sarilumab groups • **Hospital mortality**: Significantly reduced in both Tocilizumab and Sarilumab groups
Secondary Outcome/s	• **90-Day survival, Respiratory support-free days, Cardiovascular support-free days**: Significantly higher • **Progression to invasive mechanical ventilation, ECMO or death**: Significantly lower
Viva Summary	In a study comparing tocilizumab and sarilumab to standard care for critically ill COVID-19 patients in the ICU, both tocilizumab and sarilumab groups showed significantly increased organ support–free days up to day 21 and reduced hospital mortality. Additionally, secondary outcomes including 90-day survival, respiratory support–free days, and cardiovascular support–free days were significantly higher in the tocilizumab and sarilumab groups, while progression to invasive mechanical ventilation, ECMO, or death was significantly lower.
Study Conclusion	'In critically ill patients with Covid-19 receiving organ support in ICUs, treatment with the interleukin-6 receptor antagonists tocilizumab and sarilumab improved outcomes, including survival.'

REMAP-CAP (2021) IL-6: The REMAP-CAP Investigators. Interleukin-6 receptor antagonists in critically ill patients with Covid-19. N Engl J Med. 2021;384(16):1491–1502.

Study Name	RECOVERY (2022) Casirivimab/Imdevimab
Population	Hospitalised COVID-19 patients
Intervention	REGEN-COV (casirivimab/imdevimab infusion) vs standard care
Primary Outcome/s	• **28-Day mortality**: Significantly decreased in the REGEN-COV group only in seronegative patients (no detectable SARS-CoV-2 antibodies) • No significant difference in 28-day mortality when tested in the overall population (which included those with and without detectable SARS-CoV-2 antibodies)
Secondary Outcome/s	• **Progression to non-invasive or invasive ventilation**: Significantly lower in seronegative patients • **Discharged alive from hospital at 28 days**: Significantly higher in seronegative patients • In the overall population, when these secondary outcomes were tested, there were no significant differences
Viva Summary	In a study comparing the use of REGEN-COV (casirivimab/imdevimab infusion) with standard care for COVID-19 patients, it was found that 28-day mortality significantly decreased only in the REGEN-COV group among patients without detectable SARS-CoV-2 antibodies (seronegative). However, there was no significant difference in 28-day mortality across the entire population, which included both seronegative and seropositive patients. Secondary outcomes, such as progression to ventilation and discharge alive from the hospital at 28 days, also showed significant improvements in seronegative patients but not in the overall population.
Study Conclusion	'In patients admitted to hospital with COVID-19, the monoclonal antibody combination of casirivimab and imdevimab reduced 28-day mortality in patients who were seronegative (and therefore had not mounted their own humoral immune response) at baseline but not in those who were seropositive at baseline.'

RECOVERY (2022) Casirivimab/imdevimab: RECOVERY Collaborative Group. Casirivimab and imdevimab in patients admitted to hospital with COVID 19 (RECOVERY): a randomised, controlled, open-label, platform trial. Lancet. 2022;399(10325):665–676.

Study Name	RECOVERY (2022) Baricitinib
Population	Hospitalised COVID-19 patients
Intervention	Baricitinib vs usual care
Primary Outcome/s	• **28-Day mortality**: Significantly reduced in the baricitinib group (13% proportional reduction in mortality)
Secondary Outcome/s	• In the broader context of JAK inhibitors, including results from the RECOVERY trial and previous trials, there was a 20% proportional reduction in mortality, exceeding the 13% proportional reduction observed in this trial's 28-day mortality • **Death or infection due to non–COVID-19 causes, Incidence of thrombosis**: No significant difference
Viva Summary	In a study comparing baricitinib with usual care for hospitalised COVID-19 patients, there was a significant 13% reduction in 28-day mortality in the baricitinib group. Additionally, when considering other JAK inhibitors, there was a 20% reduction in mortality, surpassing the 13% reduction observed in this trial's 28-day mortality. There were no significant increases in death or infection due to non-COVID-19 causes and no significant increase in thrombosis.
Study Conclusion	'In patients hospitalised with COVID-19, baricitinib significantly reduced the risk of death but the size of benefit was somewhat smaller than that suggested by previous trials. The total randomised evidence to date suggests that JAK inhibitors (chiefly baricitinib) reduce mortality in patients hospitalised for COVID-19 by about one-fifth.'

RECOVERY (2022) Baricitinib: RECOVERY Collaborative Group. Baricitinib in patients admitted to hospital with COVID-19 (RECOVERY): a randomised, controlled, open-label, platform trial and updated meta-analysis. Lancet. 2022;400(10349):359–368.

PULMONARY EMBOLISM

Study Name	MOPETT (2013)
Population	Patients with moderate PE
Intervention	Addition of low-dose thrombolysis vs anticoagulation alone
Primary Outcome/s	• **Pulmonary hypertension on echocardiography at 28 months**: Significantly lower in low-dose thrombolysis group
Secondary Outcome/s	• **Composite of pulmonary hypertension and recurrent PE at 28 months**: Significantly lower in low-dose thrombolysis group • **Recurrent PE, Mortality, Bleeding**: No significant difference
Viva Summary	In a study comparing low-dose thrombolysis to anticoagulation alone for patients with moderate PE, the low-dose thrombolysis group showed significantly lower rates of pulmonary hypertension on echocardiography and a composite of pulmonary hypertension and recurrent PE at 28 months. However, there were no significant differences in recurrent PE, mortality, or bleeding between the two groups.
Study Conclusion	'The results from the present prospective randomized trial suggests that "safe dose" thrombolysis is safe and effective in the treatment of moderate PE, with a significant immediate reduction in the pulmonary artery pressure that was maintained at 28 months.'

MOPETT (2013): Sharifi M, Bay C, Skrocki L, et al. Moderate pulmonary embolism treated with thrombolysis (from the "MOPETT" Trial). Am J Cardiol. 2013;111(2):273–277.

Study Name	PEITHO (2014)
Population	Patients with intermediate-risk PE
Intervention	Addition of tenecteplase vs heparin alone
Primary Outcome/s	• **7-Day composite of death and haemodynamic decompensation**: Significantly lower in Tenecteplase group
Secondary Outcome/s	• **Haemodynamic decompensation**: Significantly lower in Tenecteplase group • **Major haemorrhagic stroke and major extracranial bleeding**: Significantly higher in Tenecteplase group • **7-Day and 30-Day mortality**: No significant difference
Viva Summary	In a study involving intermediate-risk pulmonary embolism patients, the addition of tenecteplase to heparin was compared to heparin alone. The primary outcome, a 7-day composite of death and haemodynamic decompensation, was significantly lower in the tenecteplase group. However, the tenecteplase group had a significantly higher incidence of major haemorrhagic stroke and major extracranial bleeding, while 7-day and 30-day mortality showed no significant difference between the two groups.
Study Conclusion	'In patients with intermediate-risk pulmonary embolism, fibrinolytic therapy prevented hemodynamic decompensation but increased the risk of major hemorrhage and stroke.'

PEITHO (2014): Meyer G, Vicaut E, Danays T, et al. Fibrinolysis for patients with intermediate-risk pulmonary embolism. N Engl J Med. 2014;370(15): 1402–1411.

VIDEO LARYNGOSCOPY

Study Name	DEVICE (2023)
Population	Critically ill adults undergoing tracheal intubation
Intervention	Videolaryngoscope (VL) vs direct laryngoscope (DL)
Primary Outcome/s	• **Successful intubation on first attempt**: Significantly higher in VL group
Secondary Outcome/s	• **Occurrence of severe complications**: No significant difference
Viva Summary	In a study comparing VL to DL for tracheal intubation in critically ill adults, the VL group had a significantly higher success rate on the first attempt. However, there was no significant difference in the occurrence of severe complications between the two groups.
Study Conclusion	'Among critically ill adults undergoing tracheal intubation in an emergency department or ICU, the use of a video laryngoscope resulted in a higher incidence of successful intubation on the first attempt than the use of a direct laryngoscope.'

DEVICE (2023): Prekker ME, Driver BE, Trent SA, Resnick-Ault D et al. Video versus direct laryngoscopy for tracheal intubation of critically ill adults. N Engl J Med. 2023 Aug 3;389(5):418–429.

OUT-OF-HOSPITAL CARDIAC ARREST (OHCA)

Study Name	TAME (2023)
Population	Patients resuscitated from out-of-hospital cardiac arrest (OHCA)
Intervention	Targeted therapeutic mild hypercapnia ($PaCO_2$ 50–55 mmHg) vs normocapnia ($PaCO_2$ 35–45 mmHg)
Primary Outcome/s	• **Favourable neurological outcome at 6 months (GOS-E score ≥5)**: No significant difference
Secondary Outcome/s	• **Poor functional outcome at 6 months, Death at ICU discharge, Death within 6 months, Adverse events**: No significant difference
Viva Summary	In a study comparing therapeutic mild hypercapnia ($PaCO_2$ 50–55 mmHg) to normocapnia ($PaCO_2$ 35–45 mmHg) in patients resuscitated from an OHCA, there was no significant difference in favourable neurological outcomes at 6 months (GOS-E score ≥5) or in secondary outcomes such as poor functional outcome at 6 months, death at ICU discharge, death within 6 months, or adverse events.
Study Conclusion	'In patients with coma who were resuscitated after out-of-hospital cardiac arrest, targeted mild hypercapnia did not lead to better neurologic outcomes at 6 months than targeted normocapnia.'

TAME (2023): Eastwood G, Nichol AD, Hodgson C, et al.; TAME Study Investigators. Mild hypercapnia or normocapnia after out-of-hospital cardiac arrest. N Engl J Med. 2023 Jul 6;389(1):45–57.

RIB FIXATION

Study Name	Dehghan et al. (2022)
Population	Patients with displaced rib fractures and flail chest or severe chest wall deformity due to blunt chest wall trauma
Intervention	Operative fixation (within 96 hours of injury) vs non-operative standard care (pain management, chest physiotherapy, ventilation as needed)
Primary Outcome/s	• **VFDs to day-28**: No significant difference
Secondary Outcome/s	• **In-hospital mortality**: Significantly higher in the non-operative group • **Rates of complications (e.g. pneumonia, VAP, sepsis, tracheostomy), Hospital/ICU LOS**: No significant difference • Subgroup analysis comparing mechanically ventilated patients at randomisation to non-ventilated ones favoured rib fixation, with an increase in VFDs and a reduction in hospital LOS
Viva Summary	In a study that compared operative fixation within 96 hours of injury with non-operative care for patients with displaced rib fractures and chest deformity from blunt chest trauma, there was no significant difference in VFDs at day 28 between the groups. However, in-hospital mortality was significantly higher in the non-operative group. The rates of complications and hospital/ICU LOS were not significantly different overall, but subgroup analysis favoured rib fixation for mechanically ventilated patients, leading to increased VFDs and reduced hospital LOS.
Study Conclusion	'The findings of this randomized clinical trial suggest that operative treatment of patients with unstable chest wall injuries has modest benefit compared with nonoperative treatment. However, the potential advantage was primarily noted in the subgroup of patients who were ventilated at the time of randomization. No benefit to operative treatment was found in patients who were not ventilated.'

Dehghan N, Nauth A, Schemitsch E, Vicente M et al.; Canadian Orthopaedic Trauma Society and the Unstable Chest Wall RCT Study Investigators. Operative vs nonoperative treatment of acute unstable chest wall injuries: a randomized clinical trial. JAMA Surg. 2022 Nov 1;157(11):983–990.

SUMMARY

1. **ARDSNet (2000):** In a study comparing low V_T ventilation (4–6 ml/kg) to traditional V_T (10–12 ml/kg) in patients with acute lung injury/ARDS, the low V_T strategy resulted in significantly lower 180-day mortality, more VFDs, a higher proportion breathing unaided by day 28, and more days without other organ failure.

2. **ALVEOLI (2004):** In a study involving patients with acute lung injury and ARDS, the comparison of higher PEEP and lower PEEP interventions, both adjusted according to FiO_2, with a maximum of 24 cmH_2O, showed no significant difference in primary outcome, which was mortality before discharge home while breathing unaided. Additionally, there were no significant differences in various secondary outcomes, including the ability to breathe without assistance at day 28, VFDs, days outside the ICU, barotrauma, and days without organ failure.

3. **OSCILLATE (2013):** In a study comparing HFOV to conventional PCV in patients with new-onset moderate-to-severe ARDS, the HFOV group had significantly higher in-hospital mortality despite lower rates of refractory hypoxaemia, leading to the early termination of the trial. The HFOV group also required higher use of neuromuscular blockers, midazolam, and vasoactive drugs compared to the conventional PCV group.

4. **OSCAR (2013):** In a study comparing HFOV to standard local practice in patients with ARDS, there was no significant difference in 30-day mortality between the two groups. However, the HFOV group showed significantly higher oxygenation and a longer duration of neuromuscular blockade, while other outcomes such as VFDs and ICU/hospital LOS did not differ significantly between the groups.

5. **Kacmarek et al. (2016):** In a study comparing an open lung approach (moderate-to-high levels of PEEP) to the ARDS network protocol in patients with established moderate/severe ARDS, there was no significant difference in 60-day mortality, ICU mortality, VFDs, or major adverse events. However, post-hoc analysis revealed that the open lung group exhibited a significant improvement in PaO_2/FiO_2 ratio at 24 hours and lower plateau pressure, PEEP, driving pressure, and FiO_2 requirement by day 3.

6. **PROSEVA (2013):** In a study comparing prone positioning for at least 16 hours a day for 28 days (or until improvement) versus supine positioning in patients with severe ARDS, the prone group showed significantly lower 28-day and 90-day mortality rates. There was no significant difference in adverse events between the two groups.

7. **ACURASYS (2010):** In a study involving patients with moderate-severe ARDS, the intervention of using cisatracurium for 48 hours resulted in a significantly lower adjusted 90-day mortality rate compared to placebo. However, there was no significant difference in actual 90-day mortality. Cisatracurium also led to significantly lower rates of barotrauma and PTX but increased the number of days with non-respiratory organ failure, while there was no significant difference in ICU-acquired paresis.

8. **ROSE (2019):** In a study involving patients with moderate-to-severe ARDS, a 48-hour infusion of cisatracurium showed no significant difference in 90-day mortality compared to usual care, leading to the study being prematurely stopped due to futility. However, the cisatracurium group experienced a higher occurrence of serious cardiovascular events. Other secondary outcomes, including 28-day mortality, days free from mechanical ventilation, ICU-free days, hospital-free days, ICU-acquired weakness, and long-term quality of life, showed no significant differences.

9. **Meduri et al. (2007):** In a study involving patients with early severe ARDS, the intervention of methylprednisolone infusion (1 mg/kg/day) was compared to a placebo. The primary outcome, which was a 1-point reduction in Lung Injury Score or successful extubation by day 7, was significantly better in the methylprednisolone group. Additionally, secondary outcomes, including the duration of mechanical ventilation, ICU LOS, ICU mortality, and infections, were significantly lower in the methylprednisolone group.

10. **DEXA-ARDS (2020):** In a study involving patients with moderate-severe ARDS, the use of IV dexamethasone (20 mg daily for 5 days, followed by 10 mg daily up to day 10 or until extubation) led to significantly more VFDs and significantly lower 60-day and ICU mortality compared to conventional treatment.

11. **CESAR (2009):** In a study involving adults with severe, potentially reversible respiratory failure, those transferred to a specialist centre and considered for ECMO showed significantly higher survival without severe disability at 6 months compared to those receiving conventional PCV. However, the ECMO group had a longer ICU/hospital LOS as a secondary outcome.

12. **EOLIA (2018):** In a study comparing VV-ECMO with conventional mechanical ventilation for adults with severe ARDS, there was no significant difference in 60-day mortality. However, the VV-ECMO group had a lower relative risk of 60-day treatment failure and the need for RRT, and they also required less proning compared to the conventional ventilation group.

13. **SUPERNOVA (2019):** In patients with ARDS, three CCO_2R systems (Hemolung, Novalung, Cardiohelp) achieved ultra-protective ventilation in 78% of patients at 8 hours and 82% at 24 hours. Survival rates were reported as 73% at day 28, with 62% of patients surviving to hospital discharge. Adverse events were documented in 39% of the patients.

14. **REST (2021):** In a study comparing $ECCO_2R$ to guideline-based mechanical ventilation for acute hypoxaemic respiratory failure, there was no significant difference in 90-day all-cause mortality, 28-day mortality, or ICU/hospital LOS. However, the $ECCO_2R$ group had significantly lower V_T on days 2–3 and fewer VFDs.

15. **ICU-ROX (2019):** In a study comparing conservative oxygen therapy (targeting S_aO_2 90–97%) to usual therapy (no upper limit) among mechanically ventilated ICU patients, there were no significant differences observed in VFDs or in secondary outcomes such as cognitive function, quality of life, and employment status. Subgroup analysis revealed that in cases of ischaemic hypoxic encephalopathy, mortality was significantly lower with conservative oxygen therapy, while in sepsis and other brain pathologies, mortality was significantly higher.

16. **HOT-ICU (2021):** In a study comparing conservative (8 kPa) and liberal (12 kPa) oxygenation levels for ICU patients receiving oxygen in a closed system, there was no significant difference in 90-day mortality rates. Additionally, no significant differences were observed in days alive without life support, days alive after hospital discharge, or serious adverse events.

17. **PILOT (2022):** In a study comparing different oxygen targets for patients on invasive mechanical ventilation, lower and intermediate oxygen levels (S_pO_2 90% and 94%) were found to have no significant difference in the number of days alive and ventilator-free at 28 days compared to higher oxygen levels (S_pO_2 98%). Additionally, there were no significant differences in secondary or exploratory outcomes, including in-hospital mortality at 28 days.

18. **BOX (Oxygen) (2022):** In a study involving comatose patients after cardiac arrest, a comparison was made between restrictive oxygenation (P_aO_2 9–10 kPa) and liberal oxygenation (P_aO_2 13–14 kPa). The primary outcome, which was a composite of death or discharge from the hospital with severe disability or coma within 90 days, showed no significant difference between the two groups. Additionally, secondary outcomes such as death within 90 days, acute kidney injury with RRT, CPC at 90 days, Montreal Cognitive Assessment score at 90 days, and neuron-specific enolase at 48 hours also did not show any significant differences.

19. **TracMan (2013):** In a study involving adults who were mechanically ventilated and at high risk of requiring prolonged ventilation, the timing of tracheostomy insertion—either early (within 4 days) or late (after 10 days, if still required)—was compared. The primary outcome, 30-day all-cause mortality, showed no significant difference between the two groups. Additionally, there were no significant differences in secondary outcomes, including survival, duration of mechanical ventilation, ICU LOS, and antibiotic use. However, survivors in the early tracheostomy group experienced significantly fewer sedation days at 30 days compared to those in the late group.

20. **Hernández et al. (2016):** In a study comparing HFNO to conventional oxygen therapy for 24 hours after extubation in low-risk patients, the HFNO group had significantly fewer cases of reintubation within 72 hours and lower rates of post-extubation respiratory failure. However, there was no significant difference in the time to reintubation between the two groups.

21. **Subirà et al. (2019):** In a study comparing two weaning methods for adults on mechanical ventilation, a 30-minute 8 cmH_2O pressure support SBT resulted in significantly higher successful extubation rates after 72 hours compared to a 2-hour T-piece SBT. Additionally,

the pressure support group had significantly lower hospital/90-day mortality rates, with no significant differences in reintubation or ICU/hospital LOS observed between the two groups.

22. **3Mg (2013):** In a study involving patients with severe acute asthma, the use of IV $MgSO_4$ compared to nebulised $MgSO_4$ or a placebo did not show any significant differences in outcomes. These outcomes included hospital admission rates, breathlessness, mortality, respiratory support, hospital length of stay, HDU/ICU admission, and changes in PEFR and physiological variables.

23. **Middleton et al. (2019):** In a study involving patients with cystic fibrosis aged ≥12 years and heterozygous for the Phe508del CFTR mutation, elexacaftor–tezacaftor–ivacaftor treatment was compared to a placebo. The primary outcome, which was the absolute change in % predicted FEV_1 after 4 weeks, showed a significant improvement in the treatment group. Additionally, secondary outcomes such as exacerbations, sweat chloride concentration, and quality of life were also significantly better in the treatment group.

24. **Delclaux et al. (2000):** In a study involving patients with acute hypoxemic, non-hypercapnic respiratory insufficiency, the addition of CPAP compared to conventional oxygen therapy did not result in a significant difference in the rate of tracheal intubation, ICU LOS, or hospital mortality. While respiratory indices initially improved in the CPAP group at 1 hour, there was no significant difference after that time. The CPAP group also experienced significantly more adverse events compared to the conventional oxygen therapy group.

25. **FLORALI (2015):** In a study comparing treatments for patients with acute hypoxaemic respiratory failure, the primary outcome, the rate of tracheal intubation, showed no significant difference between HFNO, NIV, and facemask oxygen. However, secondary outcomes revealed that HFNO led to significantly lower 90-day mortality and less discomfort at 1-hour compared to the other interventions, while there were no significant differences in ICU LOS or rate of complications.

26. **CAPE COD (2023):** In a study on ICU patients with severe community-acquired pneumonia, the administration of hydrocortisone 200 mg/day for 4 days significantly reduced 28-day mortality compared to a placebo. Additionally, the hydrocortisone group had better 90-day survival and decreased rates of endotracheal intubation and

vasopressor initiation in selected subgroups. The hydrocortisone group did need a higher daily dose of insulin, but other complications such as hospital-acquired infection and GI bleeding were not significantly different.

27. **DIABOLO (2016):** A study compared critically ill COPD patients with metabolic alkalosis who were treated with acetazolamide for up to 28 days against those given a placebo. There was no significant difference in the duration of invasive ventilation between the groups. However, the acetazolamide group exhibited lower serum bicarbonate levels and fewer days with metabolic alkalosis as secondary outcomes. Weaning duration and other ICU outcomes showed no significant differences between the groups.

28. **REMAP-CAP (2020) Corticosteroid:** In a study comparing two methods of administering hydrocortisone to severe COVID-19 patients, neither the fixed-dose nor the shock-dependent approach showed a significant advantage in terms of respiratory and cardiovascular support-free days up to day 21. The trial was stopped prematurely, and various secondary outcomes, such as in-hospital mortality and ICU/hospital LOS, did not demonstrate a clear benefit of hydrocortisone treatment over standard care.

29. **RECOVERY (2021) Dexamethasone:** In a study comparing dexamethasone (6 mg daily for 10 days) to usual care in hospitalised SARS-CoV-2 patients, the dexamethasone group had significantly lower 28-day mortality rates. This effect was more pronounced in patients on mechanical ventilation or supplemental oxygen and those with symptoms lasting over 7 days requiring invasive mechanical ventilation. Additionally, dexamethasone reduced the need for mechanical ventilation, shortened hospital LOS, and lowered the composite risk of invasive mechanical ventilation and death. There was no significant difference in outcome in patients not requiring respiratory support.

30. **REMAP-CAP (2021) IL-6:** In a study comparing tocilizumab and sarilumab to standard care for critically ill COVID-19 patients on ICU, both tocilizumab and sarilumab groups showed significantly increased organ support–free days up to day 21 and reduced hospital mortality. Additionally, secondary outcomes including 90-day survival, respiratory support–free days, and cardiovascular support–free days were significantly higher in the tocilizumab and sarilumab groups, while progression to invasive mechanical ventilation, ECMO, or death was significantly lower.

31. **RECOVERY (2022) Casirivimab/Imdevimab:** In a study comparing the use of REGEN-COV (casirivimab/imdevimab infusion) with standard care for COVID-19 patients, it was found that 28-day mortality significantly decreased only in the REGEN-COV group among patients without detectable SARS-CoV-2 antibodies (seronegative). However, there was no significant difference in 28-day mortality across the entire population, which included both seronegative and seropositive patients. Secondary outcomes, such as progression to ventilation and discharge alive from the hospital at 28 days, also showed significant improvements in seronegative patients but not in the overall population.

32. **RECOVERY (2022) Baricitinib:** In a study comparing baricitinib with usual care for hospitalised COVID-19 patients, there was a significant 13% reduction in 28-day mortality in the baricitinib group. Additionally, when considering other JAK inhibitors, there was a 20% reduction in mortality, surpassing the 13% reduction observed in this trial's 28-day mortality. There were no significant increases in death or infection due to non-COVID-19 causes and no significant increase in thrombosis.

33. **MOPETT (2013):** In a study comparing low-dose thrombolysis to anticoagulation alone for patients with moderate PE, the low-dose thrombolysis group showed significantly lower rates of pulmonary hypertension on echocardiography and a composite of pulmonary hypertension and recurrent PE at 28 months. However, there were no significant differences in recurrent PE, mortality, or bleeding between the two groups.

34. **PEITHO (2014):** In a study involving intermediate-risk pulmonary embolism patients, the addition of tenecteplase to heparin was compared to heparin alone. The primary outcome, a 7-day composite of death and haemodynamic decompensation, was significantly lower in the tenecteplase group. However, the tenecteplase group had a significantly higher incidence of major haemorrhagic stroke and major extracranial bleeding, while 7-day and 30-day mortality showed no significant difference between the two groups.

35. **DEVICE (2023):** In a study comparing VL to DL for tracheal intubation in critically ill adults, the VL group had a significantly higher success rate on the first attempt. However, there was no significant difference in the occurrence of severe complications between the two groups.

36. **TAME (2023):** In a study comparing therapeutic mild hypercapnia (P_aCO_2 50–55 mmHg) to normocapnia (P_aCO_2 35–45 mmHg) in patients resuscitated from an OHCA, there was no significant difference in favourable neurological outcomes at 6 months (GOS-E score ≥5) or in secondary outcomes such as poor functional outcome at 6 months, death at ICU discharge, death within 6 months, or adverse events.

37. **Dehghan et al. (2022):** In a study that compared operative fixation within 96 hours of injury with non-operative care for patients with displaced rib fractures and chest deformity from blunt chest trauma, there was no significant difference in VFDs at day 28 between the groups. However, in-hospital mortality was significantly higher in the non-operative group. The rates of complications and hospital/ICU LOS were not significantly different overall, but subgroup analysis favoured rib fixation for mechanically ventilated patients, leading to increased VFDs and reduced hospital LOS.

FLUIDS IN CRITICAL ILLNESS

Study Name	SAFE (2004)
Population	ICU patients
Intervention	Resuscitation using 4% HAS vs 0.9% NaCl
Primary Outcome/s	• **28-Day all-cause mortality**: No significant difference
Secondary Outcome/s	• **LOS, Duration of mechanical ventilation, RRT duration**: No significant difference • **Post-hoc 28-day mortality in TBI**: Significantly higher with 4% HAS
Viva Summary	In a study comparing resuscitation with 4% HAS to 0.9% NaCl, there was no significant difference in 28-day all-cause mortality, LOS, duration of mechanical ventilation, or RRT duration. However, post-hoc analysis revealed a significantly higher 28-day mortality in TBI patients who received 4% HAS.
Study Conclusion	'In patients in the ICU, use of either 4 percent albumin or normal saline for fluid resuscitation results in similar outcomes at 28 days.'

SAFE (2004): The SAFE Study Investigators. A comparison of albumin and saline for fluid resuscitation in the intensive care unit. N Engl J Med. 2004;350(22):2247–2256.

DOI: 10.1201/9781003468738-2

Study Name	*FEAST (2011)*
Population	Paediatric patients with severe febrile illness in a resource-limited setting in Africa
Intervention	Fluid bolus (5% albumin or 0.9% saline) vs no fluid bolus
Primary Outcome/s	• **48-Hour mortality in those without severe hypotension**: Significantly higher in fluid bolus group
Secondary Outcome/s	• **4-Week mortality**: Significantly higher in fluid bolus group
Viva Summary	In a resource-limited African setting, a study compared the use of fluid bolus (5% HAS or 0.9% saline) to no fluid bolus in paediatric patients with severe febrile illness. The study found that 48-hour mortality was significantly higher in the fluid bolus group for patients without severe hypotension, and the overall 4-week mortality was also significantly higher in the fluid bolus group.
Study Conclusion	'Fluid boluses significantly increased 48-hour mortality in critically ill children with impaired perfusion in these resource-limited settings in Africa.'

FEAST (2011): Maitland K, Kiguli S, Opoka RO, et al. Mortality after fluid bolus in African children with severe infection. N Engl J Med. 2011;364(26):2483–2495.

Study Name	CHEST (2012)
Population	Critically ill patients requiring fluid resuscitation
Intervention	6% hydroxyethyl starch (HES) vs 0.9% NaCl
Primary Outcome/s	• **90-Day mortality**: No significant difference
Secondary Outcome/s	• **Renal impairment, Use of RRT, Adverse events**: Significantly higher in HES group • **Duration of mechanical ventilation, Duration of RRT**: No significant difference
Viva Summary	In a study comparing the use of 6% HES to 0.9% NaCl for fluid resuscitation in critically ill patients, there was no significant difference in 90-day mortality between the two groups. However, the HES group experienced significantly higher rates of renal impairment, use of RRT, and adverse events, while there was no significant difference in the duration of mechanical ventilation or duration of RRT.
Study Conclusion	'In patients in the ICU, there was no significant difference in 90-day mortality between patients resuscitated with 6% HES (130/0.4) or saline. However, more patients who received resuscitation with HES were treated with renal-replacement therapy.'

CHEST (2012): Myburgh JA, Finfer S, Bellomo R, et al. Hydroxyethyl starch or saline for fluid resuscitation in intensive care. N Engl J Med. 2012;367(20):1901–1911.

Study Name	SPLIT (2015)
Population	ICU patients needing crystalloid fluid therapy
Intervention	Plasma-Lyte 148 vs 0.9% NaCl
Primary Outcome/s	• **Proportion of patients with AKI within 90 days**: No significant difference
Secondary Outcome/s	• **AKI incidence, Need for RRT, ICU readmission, LOS, Mortality**: No significant difference
Viva Summary	In a study comparing Plasma-Lyte 148 and 0.9% NaCl for ICU patients requiring crystalloid fluid therapy, there was no significant difference in the proportion of patients developing AKI within 90 days or in secondary outcomes such as AKI incidence, need for RRT, ICU readmission, LOS, or mortality rates.
Study Conclusion	'Among patients receiving crystalloid fluid therapy in the ICU, use of a buffered crystalloid compared with saline did not reduce the risk of AKI. Further large randomized clinical trials are needed to assess efficacy in higher-risk populations and to measure clinical outcomes such as mortality.'

SPLIT (2015): Young P, Bailey M, Beasley R, et al. Effect of a buffered crystalloid solution vs saline on acute kidney injury among patients in the intensive care unit. JAMA. 2015;314(16):1701–1710.

Study Name	SMART (2018)
Population	Critically ill patients
Intervention	Balanced crystalloids vs 0.9% NaCl
Primary Outcome/s	• **Major Adverse Kidney Events (MAKEs)—a composite of death, new RRT, or persistent renal dysfunction—at 30 days**: Significantly lower with balanced crystalloids
Secondary Outcome/s	• **Mortality, New need for RRT, Persistent renal dysfunction, VFDs, Vasopressor-free days**: No significant difference
Viva Summary	In a study comparing balanced crystalloids to 0.9% NaCl for critically ill patients, the primary outcome of MAKEs at 30 days was significantly lower with balanced crystalloids. However, there were no significant differences in secondary outcomes such as mortality, new need for RRT, persistent renal dysfunction, VFDs, or vasopressor-free days.
Study Conclusion	'Among critically ill adults, the use of balanced crystalloids for intravenous fluid administration resulted in a lower rate of the composite outcome of death from any cause, new renal-replacement therapy, or persistent renal dysfunction than the use of saline.'

SMART (2018): Semler MW, Self WH, Wanderer JP, et al. Balanced crystalloids versus saline in critically ill adults. N Engl J Med. 2018;378(9):829–839.

Study Name	BaSICS (2021)
Population	Adult ICU patients
Intervention	Plasma-Lyte vs 0.9% NaCl; administered via slow bolus or rapid bolus if required
Primary Outcome/s	• **90-Day mortality**: No significant difference
Secondary Outcome/s	• **Day 7 SOFA Score**: Significantly lower with Plasma-Lyte • There was no significant difference in the other 17 secondary outcomes, including the rate of AKI requiring RRT within 90 days
Viva Summary	In a study comparing Plasma-Lyte and 0.9% NaCl for adult ICU patients, administered via slow or rapid bolus, there was no significant difference in 90-day mortality. However, the secondary outcome of day 7 SOFA Score was significantly lower with Plasma-Lyte, while the other secondary outcomes, including AKI requiring RRT within 90 days, were not significantly different between the intervention groups.
Study Conclusion	'Among critically ill patients requiring fluid challenges, use of a balanced solution compared with 0.9% saline solution did not significantly reduce 90-day mortality. The findings do not support the use of this balanced solution.'

BaSICS (2021): Zampieri FG, Machado FR, Biondi RS, et al. Effect of intravenous fluid treatment with a balanced solution vs 0.9% saline solution on mortality in critically ill patients: the BaSICS randomized clinical trial. JAMA. 2021;326(9):818–829.

Study Name	PLUS (2022)
Population	Adult ICU patients
Intervention	Plasma-Lyte vs 0.9% NaCl
Primary Outcome/s	• **90-Day mortality**: No significant difference
Secondary Outcome/s	• **New requirement for RRT, Days alive and free of mechanical ventilation, Use of vasoactive drugs, Serum creatinine**: No significant difference
Viva Summary	In a study comparing Plasma-Lyte and 0.9% NaCl for adult ICU patients, there was no significant difference in 90-day mortality or secondary outcomes such as need for RRT, days free of mechanical ventilation, use of vasoactive drugs, or serum creatinine levels.
Study Conclusion	'We found no evidence that the risk of death or acute kidney injury among critically ill adults in the ICU was lower with the use of BMES (balanced multielectrolyte solution) than with saline.'

PLUS (2022): Finfer S, Micallef S, Hammond N, et al. Balanced multielectrolyte solution versus saline in critically ill adults. N Engl J Med. 2022;386(9):815–826.

Study Name	PREPARE II (2022)
Population	Critically ill adult patients undergoing tracheal intubation and positive pressure ventilation
Intervention	500-ml fluid bolus vs no fluid bolus
Primary Outcome/s	• **Incidence of cardiovascular collapse**: No significant difference
Secondary Outcome/s	• **In-hospital mortality at 28 days**: No significant difference
Viva Summary	In a study involving critically ill adult patients requiring tracheal intubation and positive pressure ventilation, the administration of a 500-ml fluid bolus showed no significant difference in the incidence of cardiovascular collapse or in-hospital mortality at 28 days compared to not receiving a fluid bolus.
Study Conclusion	'Among critically ill adults undergoing tracheal intubation, administration of an intravenous fluid bolus compared with no fluid bolus did not significantly decrease the incidence of cardiovascular collapse.'

PREPARE (2022): Russell DW, Casey JD, Gibbs KW, Ghamande S et al.; PREPARE II Investigators and the Pragmatic Critical Care Research Group. Effect of fluid bolus administration on cardiovascular collapse among critically ill patients undergoing tracheal intubation: a randomized clinical trial. JAMA. 2022 Jul 19;328(3):270–279.

PULMONARY ARTERY CATHETER USE

Study Name	PAC-Man (2005)
Population	Critically ill patients
Intervention	Pulmonary artery catheter (PAC) vs no PAC
Primary Outcome/s	• **Hospital mortality**: No significant difference
Secondary Outcome/s	• **ICU/Hospital LOS, Organ support**: No significant difference • There was a 10% complication rate in the PAC group including haematoma, arterial puncture, arrhythmia, PTX, haemothorax (HTX), and lost guidewire
Viva Summary	In a study comparing the use of PAC to no PAC in critically ill patients, there was no significant difference in hospital mortality or secondary outcomes such as ICU/hospital LOS or organ support. However, the PAC group experienced a 10% complication rate, including haematoma, arterial puncture, arrhythmia, PTX, HTX, and lost guidewire.
Study Conclusion	'Our findings indicate no clear evidence of benefit or harm by managing critically ill patients with a PAC. Efficacy studies are needed to ascertain whether management protocols involving PAC use can result in improved outcomes in specific groups if these devices are not to become a redundant technology.'

PAC-Man (2005): Harvey S, Harrison DA, Singer M, et al. Assessment of the clinical effectiveness of pulmonary artery catheters in management of patients in intensive care (PAC-Man): a randomised controlled trial. Lancet. 2005; 366(9484):472–477.

MAJOR HAEMORRHAGE

Study Name	CRASH-2 (2010)
Population	Trauma with/at risk of significant haemorrhage
Intervention	Early TXA (tranexamic acid) vs placebo
Primary Outcome/s	• **Death in hospital within 4 weeks of injury**: Significantly reduced in TXA group
Secondary Outcome/s	• **Transfusion requirement, Vaso-occlusive events, Dependency**: No significant difference
Viva Summary	In a study involving trauma patients with/at risk of significant haemorrhage, the early administration of TXA significantly reduced hospital mortality within 4 weeks of injury compared to placebo. However, there was no significant difference in transfusion requirements, vaso-occlusive events, or dependency between the two groups.
Study Conclusion	'Tranexamic acid safely reduced the risk of death in bleeding trauma patients in this study. On the basis of these results, tranexamic acid should be considered for use in bleeding trauma patients.'

CRASH-2 (2010): CRASH-2 Trial Collaborators. Effects of tranexamic acid on death, vascular occlusive events, and blood transfusion in trauma patients with significant haemorrhage (CRASH-2): a randomised, placebo-controlled trial. Lancet. 2010;376(9734):23–32.

Study Name	PROPPR (2015)
Population	Severe trauma predicted to require massive transfusion
Intervention	1:1:1 ratio vs 1:1:2 control (plasma:platelets:red cells)
Primary Outcome/s	• **24-Hour mortality, 30-Day mortality**: No significant difference
Secondary Outcome/s	• No significant difference in many secondary outcomes including time to achieve haemostasis, complications, hospital/ventilator/ICU-free days, need for surgical procedures, and functional status at discharge • Post-hoc analysis found a significant reduction in death by exsanguination within the first 24 hours and a higher rate of achieving haemostasis in the intervention group compared to the control group
Viva Summary	In a study comparing a 1:1:1 ratio of plasma:platelets:red cells to a 1:1:2 ratio for severe trauma patients requiring massive transfusion, there were no significant differences in 24-hour and 30-day mortality rates. There were also no differences in various secondary outcomes including complications, time to achieve haemostasis, or functional status at discharge. However, a post-hoc analysis did reveal a significant reduction in death due to exsanguination within the first 24 hours and a higher rate of achieving haemostasis in the 1:1:1 ratio group compared to the 1:1:2 ratio group.
Study Conclusion	'Among patients with severe trauma and major bleeding, early administration of plasma, platelets, and red blood cells in a 1:1:1 ratio compared with a 1:1:2 ratio did not result in significant differences in mortality at 24 hours or at 30 days. However, more patients in the 1:1:1 group achieved haemostasis and fewer experienced death due to exsanguination by 24 hours. Even though there was an increased use of plasma and platelets transfused in the 1:1:1 group, no other safety differences were identified between the 2 groups.'

PROPPR (2015):   Holcomb JB, Tilley BC, Baraniuk S. Transfusion of plasma, platelets, and red blood cells in a 1:1:1 vs a 1:1:2 ratio and mortality in patients with severe trauma: the PROPPR randomized clinical trial. JAMA. 2015;313(5): 471–482.

Study Name	CRYOSTAT-1 (2015)
Population	Major haemorrhage in trauma
Intervention	Addition of two early pools of cryoprecipitate vs standard care
Primary Outcome/s	• **Feasibility (assessed by the percentage of subjects in the intervention arm receiving cryoprecipitate within 90 minutes)**: Achieved in 85% (median time 60 minutes)
Secondary Outcome/s	• **All-cause mortality at 28 days**: No significant difference • **Fibrinogen (Fg) concentration**: Higher in intervention arm
Viva Summary	In a study on trauma patients, the addition of two early pools of cryoprecipitate to standard care was found to be feasible, with 85% of subjects in the intervention arm receiving cryoprecipitate within 90 minutes. There was no significant difference in 28-day all-cause mortality between the intervention and standard care groups, but the intervention group had higher fibrinogen concentrations.
Study Conclusion	'Early fibrinogen supplementation using cryoprecipitate is feasible in trauma patients. This study supports the need for a definitive RCT to determine the effect of early Fg supplementation on mortality and other clinical outcomes.'

CRYOSTAT-1 (2015): Curry N, Rourke C, Davenport R, et al. Early cryoprecipitate for major haemorrhage in trauma: a randomised controlled feasibility trial. Br J Anaesth. 2015;115(1):76–83.

Study Name	ITACTIC (2020)
Population	Trauma with haemorrhagic shock
Intervention	Managing major haemorrhage guided by VHA (viscoelastic haemostatic assays) vs CCT (conventional coagulation tests)
Primary Outcome/s	• **Alive and free of massive transfusion at 24 hours**: No significant difference
Secondary Outcome/s	• There was no significant difference in any secondary outcomes • However, in a subgroup analysis of patients with severe TBI, the VHA group had a significantly reduced 28-day mortality compared to the CCT group
Viva Summary	In a study comparing the use of viscoelastic haemostatic assays (VHA) to conventional coagulation tests (CCT) in managing major haemorrhage with shock, there was no significant difference in the primary outcome of survival without massive transfusion at 24 hours. Additionally, no significant differences were observed in any secondary outcomes overall. However, in a subgroup analysis of patients with severe TBI, the VHA group showed a significantly lower 28-day mortality rate compared to the CCT group.
Study Conclusion	'There was no difference in overall outcomes between VHA- and CCT-augmented-major haemorrhage protocols.'

ITACTIC (2020): Baksaas-Aasen K, Gall LS, Stensballe J, et al. Viscoelastic haemostatic assay augmented protocols for major trauma haemorrhage (ITACTIC): a randomized, controlled trial. Intensive Care Med. 2021;47(1):49–59.

Study Name	PATCH (2023)
Population	Adult patients with major trauma at risk for trauma-induced coagulopathy (COAST score >3)
Intervention	Early administration of 1 g TXA followed by an 8-hour TXA infusion vs placebo
Primary Outcome/s	• **Survival with favourable functional outcome at 6 months**: No significant difference
Secondary Outcome/s	• **Mortality at 24 hours and 28 days**: Significantly reduced in TXA group • No significant difference in many secondary outcomes including 6-month mortality, bleeding-related deaths, vascular occlusion, incidence of sepsis, transfusion rates, fibrinogen levels, and INR at 8 and 24 hours • Post-hoc analysis showed better neurological outcomes in patients with Abbreviated Injury Scale (AIS) ≤2 in the head or neck region in the intervention group compared to the control group
Viva Summary	In a study involving adult trauma patients at risk for trauma-induced coagulopathy (COAST score >3), early administration of 1 g TXA followed by an 8-hour TXA infusion did not significantly affect survival with favourable functional outcomes at 6 months. However, the TXA group showed significantly reduced mortality at 24 hours and 28 days, and post-hoc analysis suggested better neurological outcomes for patients with an AIS ≤2 in the head or neck region. Other secondary outcomes, such as 6-month mortality and various coagulation measures, did not differ significantly between the two groups.
Study Conclusion	'Among adults with major trauma and suspected trauma-induced coagulopathy who were being treated in advanced trauma systems, prehospital administration of tranexamic acid followed by an infusion over 8 hours did not result in a greater number of patients surviving with a favourable functional outcome at 6 months than placebo.'

PATCH (2023): PATCH-Trauma Investigators and the ANZICS Clinical Trials Group; Gruen RL, Mitra B, Bernard SA, et al. Prehospital tranexamic acid for severe trauma. N Engl J Med. 2023 Jul 13;389(2):127–136.

OUT-OF-HOSPITAL CARDIAC ARREST (OHCA)

Study Name	PARAMEDIC2 (2018)
Population	OHCA
Intervention	Adrenaline as per ALS guidance vs placebo
Primary Outcome/s	• **30-Day survival**: Significantly higher in adrenaline group
Secondary Outcome/s	• **Severe neurological impairment (mRS 4–5)**: Significantly higher in adrenaline group • **Survival with favourable outcome, ICU/Hospital LOS**: No significant difference
Viva Summary	In a study comparing adrenaline to placebo for OHCA, the adrenaline group had significantly higher 30-day survival rates but also a significantly higher incidence of severe neurological impairment (mRS 4–5). There was no significant difference in survival with favourable outcomes or ICU/hospital LOS between the two groups.
Study Conclusion	'In adults with out-of-hospital cardiac arrest, the use of epinephrine resulted in a significantly higher rate of 30-day survival than the use of placebo, but there was no significant between-group difference in the rate of a favorable neurologic outcome because more survivors had severe neurologic impairment in the epinephrine group.'

PARAMEDIC2 (2018): Perkins GD, Ji C, Deakin CD, et al. A randomized trial of epinephrine in out-of-hospital cardiac arrest. N Engl J Med. 2018;379(8):711–721.

Study Name	ARREST (2020)
Population	OHCA with initial rhythm VF or pulseless VT
Intervention	Early ECMO vs conventional resuscitation
Primary Outcome/s	• **Survival to hospital discharge**: Significantly higher in early ECMO group
Secondary Outcome/s	• **6-Month survival**: Significantly higher in early ECMO group • The study was halted due to compelling evidence of ECMO's superiority, with a posterior probability of 0.9861 exceeding the predefined threshold of 0.986
Viva Summary	In a study comparing early ECMO to conventional resuscitation for OHCA patients with initial rhythm of VF or pulseless VT, the early ECMO group showed significantly higher survival rates both at hospital discharge and at the 6-month mark. The study was stopped early due to strong evidence favouring ECMO, with a posterior probability of 0.9861 exceeding the predetermined threshold of 0.986.
Study Conclusion	'Early ECMO-facilitated resuscitation for patients with OHCA and refractory ventricular fibrillation significantly improved survival to hospital discharge compared with standard ACLS treatment.'

ARREST (2020): Yannopoulos D, Bartos J, Raveendran G, et al. Advanced reperfusion strategies for patients with out-of-hospital cardiac arrest and refractory ventricular fibrillation (ARREST): a phase 2, single centre, open-label, randomised controlled trial. Lancet. 2020;396(10265):1807–1186.

Study Name	TOMAHAWK (2021)
Population	OHCA without ST-segment elevation (age >30 years)
Intervention	Immediate angiography vs delayed/selective angiography
Primary Outcome/s	• **30-Day mortality**: No significant difference
Secondary Outcome/s	• **Composite of 30-day mortality or severe neurological deficit**: Significantly higher in the immediate angiography group • **Peak troponin release, Moderate/severe bleeding, Incidence of stroke, Incidence of RRT**: No significant difference
Viva Summary	In a study of OHCA patients aged over 30 without ST-segment elevation, immediate angiography did not significantly change 30-day mortality compared to delayed/selective angiography. However, the immediate angiography group had a notably higher rate of a composite outcome involving 30-day mortality or severe neurological deficit. Other factors such as peak troponin release, bleeding, stroke, and RRT incidence exhibited no significant differences between the two groups.
Study Conclusion	'Among patients with resuscitated out-of-hospital cardiac arrest without ST-segment elevation, a strategy of performing immediate angiography provided no benefit over a delayed or selective strategy with respect to the 30-day risk of death from any cause.'

TOMAHAWK (2021): Desch S, Freund A, Akin I, et al. Angiography after out-of-hospital cardiac arrest without ST-segment elevation. N Engl J Med. 2021;385(27):2544–2553.

Study Name	BOX (Blood Pressure) (2022)
Population	Comatose survivors of an OHCA
Intervention	Higher MAP target (>77 mmHg) vs standard MAP target (>63 mmHg)
Primary Outcome/s	• **Composite of death or discharge from hospital up to day 90 with a Cerebral Performance Score of 3–4**: No significant difference
Secondary Outcome/s	• **90-Day mortality, Neuron-specific enolase levels, Adverse event rates**: No significant difference
Viva Summary	In a study involving comatose survivors of an OHCA, there was no significant difference in death or hospital discharge with a Cerebral Performance Score of 3–4 between those treated with a higher MAP target (>77 mmHg) and those with a standard MAP target (>63 mmHg) up to day 90. Additionally, there were no significant differences in secondary outcomes, including 90-day mortality, neuron-specific enolase levels, and adverse event rates.
Study Conclusion	'Targeting a mean arterial blood pressure of 77 mm Hg or 63 mm Hg in patients who had been resuscitated from cardiac arrest did not result in significantly different percentages of patients dying or having severe disability or coma.'

BOX (Blood Pressure)(2022): Kjaergaard J, Møller JE, Schmidt H, et al. Blood-pressure targets in comatose survivors of cardiac arrest. N Engl J Med. 2022 Oct 20;387(16):1456–1466.

Study Name	*INCEPTION (2023)*
Population	Patients with refractory OHCA and initial ventricular arrhythmia
Intervention	Extracorporeal cardiopulmonary resuscitation (ECPR) vs conventional CPR (CCPR)
Primary Outcome/s	• **Survival with a favourable neurologic outcome at 30 days**: No significant difference
Secondary Outcome/s	• **3-Month and 6-Month survival with a favourable neurologic outcome**: No significant difference • **Admission to ICU**: More common in the ECPR group
Viva Summary	In a study involving patients with refractory OHCA and an initial ventricular arrhythmia, the use of ECPR did not significantly improve survival with a favourable neurological outcome at 30 days compared to conventional CPR. Additionally, the ECPR group had a higher rate of admission to ICU, with no significant differences in 3-month or 6-month survival with a favourable neurological outcome.
Study Conclusion	'In patients with refractory out-of-hospital cardiac arrest, extracorporeal CPR and conventional CPR had similar effects on survival with a favourable neurologic outcome.'

INCEPTION (2023): Suverein MM, Delnoij TSR, Lorusso R, et al. Early extracorporeal CPR for refractory out-of-hospital cardiac arrest. N Engl J Med. 2023 Jan 26;388(4):299–309.

RUPTURED ABDOMINAL AORTIC ANEURYSM (AAA)

Study Name	IMPROVE (2014)
Population	Ruptured AAA
Intervention	EVAR vs open repair
Primary Outcome/s	• **30-Day mortality**: No significant difference
Secondary Outcome/s	• EVAR with local anaesthesia alone led to a four-fold reduction in 30-day mortality compared to general anaesthesia • **Permissive hypotension**: SBP <70 mmHg was independently linked to a high 30-day mortality rate of 51%
Viva Summary	In a study comparing EVAR to open repair for ruptured AAA, there was no significant difference in 30-day mortality rate between the two interventions. However, EVAR with local anaesthesia alone resulted in a four-fold reduction in 30-day mortality compared to general anaesthesia. Additionally, maintaining permissive hypotension with an SBP <70 mmHg was independently associated with a high 30-day mortality rate of 51%.
Study Conclusion	'These findings suggest that the outcome of ruptured AAA might be improved by wider use of local anaesthesia for EVAR and that a minimum blood pressure of 70 mmHg is too low a threshold for permissive hypotension.'

IMPROVE (2014): IMPROVE Trial Investigators. Observations from the IMPROVE trial concerning the clinical care of patients with ruptured abdominal aortic aneurysm. Br J Surg. 2014;101(3):216–224.

ACUTE CORONARY SYNDROME

Study Name	ISIS-2 (1988)
Population	Acute MI with 24-hour symptom onset
Intervention	Streptokinase/aspirin/both vs placebo
Primary Outcome/s	• **5-Week vascular mortality**: Significantly reduced by 25% with streptokinase alone, 23% with aspirin alone, and 40% in combination
Secondary Outcome/s	• Streptokinase increased the incidence of transfusion-requiring bleeding and cerebral haemorrhage. However, it reduced the occurrence of other types of strokes, leading to no overall increase in the total number of strokes • Aspirin reduced reinfarction and stroke rates without significantly increasing cerebral haemorrhage or transfusion-requiring bleeds • Combining streptokinase and aspirin reduced reinfarction, stroke, and death compared to receiving no treatment • The differences in vascular and all-cause mortality produced by streptokinase and aspirin remained highly significant after 15 months of follow-up.
Viva Summary	In a study comparing treatments for acute MI with 24-hour symptom onset, streptokinase alone reduced vascular mortality by 25%, aspirin alone reduced it by 23%, and the combination of both reduced it by 40% at 5 weeks. Combining streptokinase and aspirin also lowered reinfarction, stroke, and death rates compared to no treatment, and these benefits remained significant after 15 months of follow-up.
Study Conclusion	'Although further research may eventually identify some fibrinolytic or antithrombotic regimens more effective than those tested in ISIS-2, streptokinase and aspirin are practicable and are of demonstrated value and safety. If both are used widely, they should avoid several tens of thousands of deaths each year.'

ISIS-2 (1988): ISIS-2 (Second International Study of Infarct Survival) Collaborative Group. Randomised trial of intravenous streptokinase, oral aspirin, both, or neither among 17,187 cases of suspected acute myocardial infarction: ISIS-2. Lancet. 1988;2(8607):349–360.

Study Name	NORDISTEMI (2010)
Population	STEMI post-thrombolysis
Intervention	Immediate PCI vs PCI for rescue/deterioration
Primary Outcome/s	• **Composite endpoint of death, reinfarction, stroke, or new ischaemia at 1 year**: No significant difference
Secondary Outcome/s	• **The secondary composite endpoint of death, reinfarction, or stroke at 12 months**: Significantly lower in the immediate PCI group • **Bleeding, Infarct size**: No significant difference
Viva Summary	In a study comparing immediate PCI to PCI for rescue/deterioration in STEMI patients post-thrombolysis, the primary composite outcome of death, reinfarction, stroke, or new ischaemia at 1 year was not significantly different between the treatment groups. However, the secondary composite outcome of death, reinfarction, or stroke at 12 months was significantly lower in the immediate PCI group. Bleeding and infarct size were not significantly different.
Study Conclusion	'Immediate transfer for PCI did not improve the primary outcome significantly, but reduced the rate of death, reinfarction, or stroke at 12 months in patients with STEMI, treated with thrombolysis and clopidogrel in areas with long transfer distances.'

NORDISTEMI (2010): Bøhmer E, Hoffmann P, Abdelnoor M, et al. Efficacy and safety of immediate angioplasty versus ischaemia-guided management after thrombolysis in acute myocardial infarction in areas with very long transfer distances results of the NORDISTEMI (NORwegian study on DIstinct treatment of ST-elevation myocardial infarction). J Am Coll Cardiol. 2010;55(2):102–110.

BETA-BLOCKERS

Study Name	POISE (2008)
Population	Patients undergoing non-cardiac surgery
Intervention	Metoprolol succinate pre- and post-op vs placebo
Primary Outcome/s	• **Composite outcome of cardiovascular death, non-fatal MI, and non-fatal cardiac arrest at 30 days**: Significantly lower in metoprolol group
Secondary Outcome/s	• **30-Day mortality, Stroke, Clinically significant hypotension, Bradycardia**: Significantly higher in metoprolol group • **New clinically significant AF, Cardiac revascularisation**: Significantly lower in metoprolol group
Viva Summary	In a study involving patients undergoing non-cardiac surgery, those who received metoprolol succinate before and after the operation had a significantly lower rate of a composite outcome, which included cardiovascular death, non-fatal MI, and non-fatal cardiac arrest at 30 days, compared to those who received a placebo. They also had significantly lower rates of new clinically significant atrial fibrillation and the need for cardiac revascularisation. However, the metoprolol group also had significantly higher 30-day all-cause mortality, stroke, clinically significant hypotension, and bradycardia.
Study Conclusion	'Our results highlight the risk in assuming a perioperative beta-blocker regimen has benefit without substantial harm, and the importance and need for large randomised trials in the perioperative setting. Patients are unlikely to accept the risks associated with perioperative extended-release metoprolol.'

POISE (2008): POISE Study Group. Effects of extended-release metoprolol succinate in patients undergoing non-cardiac surgery (POISE trial): a randomised controlled trial. Lancet. 2008;371(9627):1839–1847.

HEART FAILURE

Study Name	SHOCK (1999)
Population	Shock due to LV failure complicating MI
Intervention	Emergency revascularisation (CABG/angioplasty) vs initial medical stabilisation
Primary Outcome/s	• **30-Day mortality**: No significant difference
Secondary Outcome/s	• **6-Month mortality**: Significantly lower in emergency revascularisation group
Viva Summary	In a study comparing emergency revascularisation (CABG/angioplasty) to initial medical stabilisation for patients with shock due to LV failure following an MI, there was no significant difference in 30-day mortality. However, the emergency revascularisation group had a significantly lower 6-month mortality rate.
Study Conclusion	'In patients with cardiogenic shock, emergency revascularization did not significantly reduce overall mortality at 30 days. However, after six months there was a significant survival benefit. Early revascularization should be strongly considered for patients with acute myocardial infarction complicated by cardiogenic shock.'

SHOCK (1999): Hochman JS, Sleeper LA, Webb JG, et al. Early revascularization in acute myocardial infarction complicated by cardiogenic shock. N Engl J Med. 1999;341(9):625–634.

Study Name	REMATCH (2001)
Population	End-stage HF
Intervention	LVAD vs medical management
Primary Outcome/s	• **All-cause mortality at 1 and 2 years**: Significantly lower in LVAD group
Secondary Outcome/s	• **Quality of life at 1 year**: Higher in LVAD group • **Serious adverse events**: Significantly higher in LVAD group (primarily related to infection, bleeding, and device malfunction)
Viva Summary	In a study comparing LVAD intervention to medical management for end-stage heart failure, the LVAD group had significantly lower all-cause mortality at 1 and 2 years and improved quality of life. However, the LVAD group also experienced significantly more serious adverse events, mainly related to infection, bleeding, and device malfunction.
Study Conclusion	'The use of a left ventricular assist device in patients with advanced heart failure resulted in a clinically meaningful survival benefit and an improved quality of life. A left ventricular assist device is an acceptable alternative therapy in selected patients who are not candidates for cardiac transplantation.'

REMATCH (2001): Rose EA, Gelijns AC, Moskowitz AJ, et al. Long-term use of a left ventricular assist device for end-stage heart failure. N Engl J Med. 2001;345(20):1435–1443.

Study Name	IABP-SHOCK II (2012)
Population	Acute MI and cardiogenic shock
Intervention	Intra-aortic balloon pump (IABP) vs medical therapy
Primary Outcome/s	• **30-Day all-cause mortality**: No significant difference
Secondary Outcome/s	• **Re-infarction, Peripheral ischaemia, Bleeding, Sepsis**: No significant difference
Viva Summary	In a study comparing the use of an IABP to medical therapy for patients with an acute MI and cardiogenic shock, there was no significant difference in 30-day all-cause mortality or secondary outcomes including reinfarction, peripheral ischaemia, bleeding, or sepsis.
Study Conclusion	'The use of intraaortic balloon counterpulsation did not significantly reduce 30-day mortality in patients with cardiogenic shock complicating acute myocardial infarction for whom an early revascularization strategy was planned.'

IABP-SHOCK II (2012): Thiele H, Zeymer U, Neumann FJ, et al. Intraaortic balloon support for myocardial infarction with cardiogenic shock. N Engl J Med. 2012;367(14):1287–1296.

Study Name	ECMO-CS (2022)
Population	Patients with rapidly deteriorating or severe cardiogenic shock
Intervention	Immediate initiation of VA-ECMO vs initial conservative therapy
Primary Outcome/s	• **Composite outcome of death, resuscitated cardiac arrest, or commencement of another mechanical circulatory support at 30 days**: No significant difference
Secondary Outcome/s	No significant differences in any of the predefined secondary outcomes or serious adverse events were observed
Viva Summary	In a study comparing the use of immediate VA-ECMO versus conservative therapy in patients with severe cardiogenic shock, there was no significant difference in the composite outcome of death, resuscitated cardiac arrest, or the need for another mechanical circulatory support at 30 days. Additionally, no significant differences were observed in secondary outcomes or serious adverse events.
Study Conclusion	'Immediate implementation of VA-ECMO in patients with rapidly deteriorating or severe cardiogenic shock did not improve clinical outcomes compared with an early conservative strategy that permitted downstream use of VA-ECMO in case of worsening hemodynamic status.'

ECMO-CS (2022): Ostadal P, Rokyta R, Karasek J, et al. Extracorporeal membrane oxygenation in the therapy of cardiogenic shock: results of the ECMO-CS randomized clinical trial. Circulation. 2023 Feb 7;147(6):454–464

VASOPRESSOR WEANING

Study Name	MIDAS (2020)
Population	Adults > 18 years on single agent vasopressors unable to be liberated from vasopressors for > 24 hours
Intervention	Midodrine 20 mg orally every 8 hours vs placebo
Primary Outcome/s	• **Time to vasopressor discontinuation**: No significant difference • Post-hoc subgroup analysis showed that midodrine significantly reduced vasopressor discontinuation times in patients with epidural analgesia
Secondary Outcome/s	• **Readiness for ICU discharge, ICU/Hospital LOS, ICU readmission**: No significant difference • **Bradycardia**: Significantly higher in midodrine group
Viva Summary	In a study comparing 20 mg of midodrine administered every 8 hours to a placebo in adults on single-agent vasopressors, no significant difference was found in the overall time to vasopressor discontinuation. However, a post-hoc analysis showed a significant reduction in discontinuation time among patients with epidural analgesia. Secondary outcomes, including readiness for ICU discharge, ICU/hospital LOS, and ICU readmission rates, showed no significant differences. Notably, bradycardia rates were significantly higher in the midodrine group.
Study Conclusion	'Midodrine did not accelerate liberation from intravenous vasopressors and was not effective for the treatment of hypotension in critically ill patients.'

MIDAS (2020): Santer P, Anstey MH, Patrocínio MD, Wibrow B, et al.; MIDAS Study Group. Effect of midodrine versus placebo on time to vasopressor discontinuation in patients with persistent hypotension in the intensive care unit (MIDAS): an international randomised clinical trial. Intensive Care Med. 2020 Oct;46(10):1884–1893.

FLUIDS IN SEPSIS

Study Name	6S (2012)
Population	Critically ill adults with severe sepsis
Intervention	6% HES vs Ringer's acetate
Primary Outcome/s	• **Death or Dialysis dependence at 90 days**: Significantly higher in HES group
Secondary Outcome/s	• **RRT use**: Significantly higher in HES group
Viva Summary	In a study comparing the use of 6% HES to Ringer's acetate in critically ill adults with severe sepsis, the HES group had significantly higher rates of death or dialysis dependence at 90 days, as well as a significantly higher use of RRT compared to the Ringer's acetate group.
Study Conclusion	'Patients with severe sepsis assigned to fluid resuscitation with HES 130/0.42 had an increased risk of death at day 90 and were more likely to require renal-replacement therapy, as compared with those receiving Ringer's acetate.'

6S (2012): Perner A, Haase N, Guttormsen AB, et al. Hydroxyethyl starch 130/0.42 versus Ringer's acetate in severe sepsis. N Engl J Med. 2012; 367(2):124–134.

Study Name	ALBIOS (2014)
Population	Adults with severe sepsis or septic shock
Intervention	20% HAS and crystalloid (with a target serum albumin ≥30 g/l) vs crystalloid only
Primary Outcome/s	• **28-Day mortality**: No significant difference
Secondary Outcome/s	• **90-Day mortality**: No significant difference
Viva Summary	In a study involving adults with severe sepsis or septic shock, administering 20% HAS along with crystalloid to maintain a target serum albumin level of ≥30 g/l did not lead to a significant difference in 28-day or 90-day mortality when compared to the use of crystalloid alone.
Study Conclusion	'In patients with severe sepsis, albumin replacement in addition to crystalloids, as compared with crystalloids alone, did not improve the rate of survival at 28 and 90 days.'

ALBIOS (2014): Caironi P, Tognoni G, Masson S, et al. Albumin replacement in patients with severe sepsis or septic shock. N Engl J Med. 2014;370(15):1412–1421.

Study Name	CLASSIC (2022)
Population	Adult patients in ICU with septic shock
Intervention	Restrictive fluid therapy vs standard care
Primary Outcome/s	• **90-Day mortality**: No significant difference
Secondary Outcome/s	• **Serious adverse events, Days alive without life support, Days alive and out of the hospital**: No significant difference
Viva Summary	In a study involving adult ICU patients with septic shock, a comparison was made between restrictive fluid therapy and standard care. The primary outcome of 90-day mortality was not significantly different between the two groups. Similarly, secondary outcomes, including serious adverse events, days alive without life support, and days alive and out of the hospital were not significantly different.
Study Conclusion	'Among adult patients with septic shock in the ICU, intravenous fluid restriction did not result in fewer deaths at 90 days than standard intravenous fluid therapy.'

CLASSIC (2022): Meyhoff TS, Hjortrup PB, Wetterslev J, et al.; CLASSIC Trial Group. Restriction of intravenous fluid in ICU patients with septic shock. N Engl J Med. 2022 Jun 30;386(26):2459–2470.

CIRCULATORY SUPPORT IN SEPSIS

Study Name	VASST (2008)
Population	Septic shock
Intervention	Vasopressin 0.01–0.03 units/min vs norepinephrine (NA) 5–15 µg/min
Primary Outcome/s	• **28-Day mortality**: No significant difference
Secondary Outcome/s	• **90-Day mortality, Need for RRT, LOS, Organ dysfunction, Adverse events**: No significant difference • **Norepinephrine infusion rate**: Significantly lower in vasopressin group • **Post-hoc analysis**: There may be a possible advantage of vasopressin in patients with less severe shock
Viva Summary	In a study comparing vasopressin at 0.01–0.03 units/min to norepinephrine at 5–15 µg/min for septic shock, there was no significant difference in 28-day mortality or various secondary outcomes, including 90-day mortality, need for RRT, LOS, organ dysfunction, and adverse events. However, the vasopressin group did have a significantly lower norepinephrine infusion rate, and a post-hoc analysis suggested a potential advantage of vasopressin in patients with less severe shock.
Study Conclusion	'Low-dose vasopressin did not reduce mortality rates as compared with norepinephrine among patients with septic shock who were treated with catecholamine vasopressors.'

VASST (2008): Russell JA, Walley KR, Singer J, et al. Vasopressin versus norepinephrine infusion in patients with septic shock. N Engl J Med. 2008;358(9): 877–887.

Study Name	SOAP II (2010)
Population	Patients with circulatory shock
Intervention	Dopamine vs noradrenaline (NA)
Primary Outcome/s	• **28-Day mortality**: No significant difference
Secondary Outcome/s	• **Death from refractory shock, Incidence of arrhythmias, 28-day mortality in cardiogenic shock**: Significantly higher with dopamine • **Days without vasopressor**: Significantly lower with dopamine • **Days without ICU care, Days without organ support**: No significant difference
Viva Summary	In a study comparing the use of dopamine and noradrenaline in patients with circulatory shock, there was no significant difference in 28-day mortality. However, dopamine was associated with fewer vasopressor-free days, higher rates of death from refractory shock, increased arrhythmias, and higher 28-day mortality in cardiogenic shock. There were no significant differences in days without ICU care or days without organ support.
Study Conclusion	'Although there was no significant difference in the rate of death between patients with shock who were treated with dopamine as the first-line vasopressor agent and those who were treated with norepinephrine, the use of dopamine was associated with a greater number of adverse events.'

SOAP II (2010): De Backer D, Biston P, Devriendt J, et al. Comparison of dopamine and norepinephrine in the treatment of shock. N Engl J Med. 2010;362(9):779–789.

Study Name	VANISH (2016)
Population	Adult patients with septic shock requiring vasopressors despite fluid resuscitation
Intervention	Patients were randomised into one of four treatment groups: 1. Vasopressin + hydrocortisone 2. Vasopressin + placebo 3. Noradrenaline + hydrocortisone 4. Noradrenaline + placebo
Primary Outcome/s	• **Kidney failure–free days during the 28-day period**: No significant difference
Secondary Outcome/s	• **Rates of RRT**: Lower in vasopressin groups • No significant differences were observed between the groups in other secondary outcomes, including mortality rates, renal failure rate, use of inotropes, shock reversal, SOFA scores, duration of mechanical ventilation, ICU and hospital LOS, and serious adverse events
Viva Summary	In a study involving adult patients with septic shock requiring vasopressors despite fluid resuscitation, four treatment groups were compared: 1) vasopressin + hydrocortisone, 2) vasopressin + placebo, 3) noradrenaline + hydrocortisone, and 4) noradrenaline + placebo. The primary outcome of kidney failure–free days during the 28-day period was not significantly different between the groups. Analysis of secondary outcomes revealed no significant differences in outcomes such as mortality rates, kidney failure rates, or SOFA scores, but did show lower rates of RRT in the vasopressin groups.
Study Conclusion	'Among adults with septic shock, the early use of vasopressin compared with norepinephrine did not improve the number of kidney failure–free days. Although these findings do not support the use of vasopressin to replace norepinephrine as initial treatment in this situation, the confidence interval included a potential clinically important benefit for vasopressin, and larger trials may be warranted to assess this further.'

VANISH (2016): Gordon AC, Mason AJ, Thirunavukkarasu N, et al.; VANISH Investigators. Effect of early vasopressin vs norepinephrine on kidney failure in patients with septic shock: the VANISH randomized clinical trial. JAMA. 2016 Aug 2;316(5):509–18.

Study Name	LeoPARDS (2016)
Population	Adults with sepsis
Intervention	Levosimendan vs placebo
Primary Outcome/s	• **Mean daily SOFA Score up to day 28**: No significant difference
Secondary Outcome/s	• **28-Day mortality**: No significant difference • **Time to weaning from mechanical ventilation**: Lower likelihood of successful weaning in the levosimendan group over 28 days • **Risk of supraventricular tachyarrhythmia**: Higher in levosimendan group
Viva Summary	In a study comparing levosimendan to a placebo for adults with sepsis, there was no difference in mean daily SOFA Score up to day 28. However, the levosimendan group had a lower likelihood of successful weaning from mechanical ventilation over 28 days and a higher risk of supraventricular tachyarrhythmias. There was no significant difference in 28-day mortality.
Study Conclusion	'The addition of levosimendan to standard treatment in adults with sepsis was not associated with less severe organ dysfunction or lower mortality. Levosimendan was associated with a lower likelihood of successful weaning from mechanical ventilation and a higher risk of supraventricular tachyarrhythmia.'

LeoPARDS (2016): Gordon AC, Perkins GD, Singer M, et al. Levosimendan for the prevention of acute organ dysfunction in sepsis. N Engl J Med. 2016 Oct 27;375(17):1638–1648.

Study Name	CLOVERS (2023)
Population	Adult patients with sepsis-induced hypotension
Intervention	Restrictive fluid strategy (with early vasopressor use) vs liberal fluid strategy (with later vasopressor use)
Primary Outcome/s	• **All-cause mortality before discharge home by day 90**: No significant difference
Secondary Outcome/s	• No significant differences were observed in various outcomes, such as organ support therapy, ventilator use, ICU-free days, intubation, ARDS onset, or serious adverse events • The restrictive fluid group had a higher rate of ICU admissions during the initial 7 days on post-hoc analysis
Viva Summary	In a study involving adult sepsis patients with hypotension, a comparison was made between a restrictive fluid strategy with early vasopressor use and a liberal fluid strategy with later vasopressor use. The primary outcome of all-cause mortality before discharge was not significantly different between the two strategies at 90 days. Additionally, there were no significant differences in secondary outcomes, except for a higher rate of ICU admissions in the restrictive fluid group during the initial 7 days on post-hoc analysis.
Study Conclusion	'Among patients with sepsis-induced hypotension, the restrictive fluid strategy that was used in this trial did not result in significantly lower (or higher) mortality before discharge home by day 90 than the liberal fluid strategy.'

CLOVERS (2023): National Heart, Lung, and Blood Institute Prevention and Early Treatment of Acute Lung Injury Clinical Trials Network; Shapiro NI, Douglas IS, Brower RG, et al. Early restrictive or liberal fluid management for sepsis-induced hypotension. N Engl J Med. 2023 Feb 9;388(6):499–510.

RESUSCITATION TARGETS IN SEPSIS

Study Name	TRISS (2014)
Population	Patients with septic shock
Intervention	Transfusion threshold ≤70 g/l (lower) vs ≤90 g/l (higher)
Primary Outcome/s	• **90-Day mortality**: No significant difference
Secondary Outcome/s	• **Median number of transfusions**: Significantly lower in the lower threshold transfusion group • **Patients not undergoing transfusion**: Significantly higher in the lower threshold transfusion group
Viva Summary	In a study involving patients with septic shock, two transfusion thresholds were compared: ≤70 g/l (lower) and ≤90 g/l (higher). There was no significant difference in 90-day mortality between the groups. However, the lower threshold group required significantly fewer transfusions and a higher proportion of patients did not undergo any transfusion at all compared to the higher threshold group.
Study Conclusion	'Among patients with septic shock, mortality at 90 days and rates of ischemic events and use of life support were similar among those assigned to blood transfusion at a higher hemoglobin threshold and those assigned to blood transfusion at a lower threshold; the latter group received fewer transfusions.'

TRISS (2014): Holst LB, Haase N, Wetterslev J, et al. Lower versus higher hemoglobin threshold for transfusion in septic shock. N Engl J Med. 2014;371(15):1381–1391.

Study Name	SEPSISPAM (2014)
Population	Patients with septic shock
Intervention	Higher MAP target (80–85 mmHg) vs lower MAP target (65–70 mmHg)
Primary Outcome/s	• **28-Day mortality**: No significant difference

Secondary Outcome/s	• **90-Day mortality, Serious adverse events**: No significant difference
	• **New Atrial Fibrillation (AF)**: Significantly higher rates in the 80–85 mmHg target group
	• Subgroup analysis in patients with chronic hypertension:
	  – High MAP group had significantly less serum creatinine doubling compared to the low MAP group
	  – High MAP group also required RRT significantly less frequently from day 1 to 7 than the low MAP group

Viva Summary	In a study involving patients with septic shock, a comparison was made between two MAP targets: a higher target of 80–85 mmHg and a lower target of 65–70 mmHg. There was no difference in 28-day mortality between the two groups. Similarly, there were no significant differences in 90-day mortality or serious adverse events. However, the 80–85 mmHg target group had a significantly higher rate of new AF. Subgroup analysis in patients with chronic hypertension revealed that the high MAP group required RRT less frequently from day 1 to 7 compared to the lower MAP group.
Study Conclusion	'Targeting a mean arterial pressure of 80 to 85 mm Hg, as compared with 65 to 70 mm Hg, in patients with septic shock undergoing resuscitation did not result in significant differences in mortality at either 28 or 90 days.'

SEPSISPAM (2014): Asfar P, Meziani F, Hamel J. High versus low blood-pressure target in patients with septic shock. N Engl J Med. 2014;370(17): 1583–1593.

Study Name	ANDROMEDA-SHOCK (2019)
Population	Patients with septic shock
Intervention	Resuscitation aiming to normalise capillary refill time (CRT) vs decreasing lactate levels, during an 8-hour period
Primary Outcome/s	• **28-Day mortality**: No significant difference
Secondary Outcome/s	• **Organ dysfunction at 72 hours**: Significantly lower with CRT normalisation group • **90-Day mortality, Organ support–free days (mechanical ventilation, RRT, vasopressors), LOS**: No significant difference
Viva Summary	In a study involving patients with septic shock, there was no significant difference in 28-day mortality between those receiving resuscitation to normalise capillary refill time and those aiming to decrease lactate levels over an 8-hour period. However, the group focused on capillary refill time normalisation exhibited significantly lower organ dysfunction at 72 hours. Secondary outcomes such as 90-day mortality, organ support-free days, and LOS were not significantly different between the two intervention groups.
Study Conclusion	'Among patients with septic shock, a resuscitation strategy targeting normalization of capillary refill time, compared with a strategy targeting serum lactate levels, did not reduce all-cause 28-day mortality.'

ANDROMEDA-SHOCK (2019): Hernández G, Ospina-Tascón GA, Damani LP, et al. Effect of a resuscitation strategy targeting peripheral perfusion status vs serum lactate levels on 28-day mortality among patients with septic shock: the ANDROMEDA-SHOCK randomized clinical trial. JAMA. 2019;321(7): 654–664.

Study Name	65 (2020)
Population	Patients >65 years of age with vasodilatory hypotension, recently started on vasopressors
Intervention	Permissive hypotension (MAP 60–65 mmHg) vs standard care
Primary Outcome/s	• **90-Day mortality**: No significant difference
Secondary Outcome/s	• **Vasopressor exposure**: Significantly lower exposure to vasopressors in permissive hypotension group • **ICU/Hospital mortality, Duration of organ support, LOS, Cognitive decline, Quality of life**: No significant difference • Subgroup analysis indicated greater survival benefits in chronically hypertensive patients within the permissive hypotension group and a trend towards improved survival with increasing age
Viva Summary	In a study involving patients over 65 years with vasodilatory hypotension who were initiated on vasopressors, a comparison was made between permissive hypotension (targeting a MAP of 60–65 mmHg) and standard care. Ninety-day mortality was not significantly different between the two groups; however, the permissive hypotension group had significantly lower exposure to vasopressors. Other secondary outcomes, such as ICU/hospital mortality, duration of organ support, LOS, cognitive decline, and quality of life, were not significantly different. Subgroup analysis suggested potential survival benefits for chronically hypertensive patients in the permissive hypotension group and a possible trend towards improved survival with increasing age.
Study Conclusion	'Among patients 65 years or older receiving vasopressors for vasodilatory hypotension, permissive hypotension compared with usual care did not result in a statistically significant reduction in mortality at 90 days. However, the confidence interval around the point estimate for the primary outcome should be considered when interpreting the clinical importance of the study.'

65 (2020): Lamontagne F, Richards-Belle A, Thomas K, et al. Effect of reduced exposure to vasopressors on 90-day mortality in older critically ill patients with vasodilatory hypotension: a randomized clinical trial. JAMA. 2020;323(10):938–949.

EARLY GOAL-DIRECTED THERAPY (EGDT) IN SEPSIS

Study Name	Rivers et al. (2001)
Population	Patients with severe sepsis or septic shock
Intervention	EGDT vs standard care
Primary Outcome/s	• **In-hospital mortality**: Significantly lower with EGDT
Secondary Outcome/s	• **Sepsis Severity**: Significantly reduced with EGDT • **Mortality at 28 and 60 days**: Significantly lower with EGDT
Viva Summary	In a study involving patients with severe sepsis or septic shock, EGDT was compared to standard care. The results showed that EGDT led to significantly lower in-hospital mortality, reduced severity of sepsis, and lower mortality rates at 28 and 60 days.
Study Conclusion	'Early goal-directed therapy provides significant benefits with respect to outcome in patients with severe sepsis and septic shock.'

River E, Nguyen B, Havstad S, et al. Early goal-directed therapy in the treatment of severe sepsis and septic shock. N Engl J Med. 2001;345(19): 1368–1377.

Study Name	ARISE (2014)
Population	Patients with septic shock
Intervention	EGDT vs standard care
Primary Outcome/s	• **90-Day all-cause mortality**: No significant difference
Secondary Outcome/s	• **Vasopressor and red cell transfusion use**: Significantly higher with EGDT • **ED/Hospital LOS, Duration on vasopressors, RRT, Mechanical ventilation**: No significant difference
Viva Summary	In a study comparing EGDT to standard care for patients with septic shock, there was no significant difference in 90-day all-cause mortality. However, the use of vasopressors and red cell transfusions was significantly higher in the EGDT group. Other secondary outcomes, including ED/hospital LOS, duration of time on vasopressors, RRT, and mechanical ventilation, were not significantly different between the two groups.
Study Conclusion	'In critically ill patients presenting to the emergency department with early septic shock, EGDT did not reduce all-cause mortality at 90 days.'

ARISE (2014): The ARISE Investigators and the ANZICS Clinical Trials Group. Goal-directed resuscitation for patients with early septic shock. N Engl J Med. 2014;371(16):1496–1506.

Study Name	ProCESS (2014)
Population	Patients with sepsis
Intervention	6 Hours of EGDT vs protocol-guided standard care vs usual care
Primary Outcome/s	• **60-Day mortality**: No significant difference
Secondary Outcome/s	• **90-Day mortality, 1-Year mortality**: No significant difference
Viva Summary	In a study comparing the treatment of patients with sepsis, three interventions were examined: 6 hours of EGDT, protocol-guided standard care, and usual care. The primary outcome, 60-day mortality, was not significantly different between the three groups. Similarly, there were no significant differences in secondary outcomes including 90-day mortality and 1-year mortality.
Study Conclusion	'In a multicenter trial conducted in the tertiary care setting, protocol-based resuscitation of patients in whom septic shock was diagnosed in the emergency department did not improve outcomes.'

ProCESS (2014): The ProCESS Investigators. A randomized trial of protocol-based care for early septic shock. N Engl J Med. 2014;370(18):1683–1693.

Study Name	ProMISe (2015)
Population	Patients with septic shock
Intervention	EGDT vs standard care
Primary Outcome/s	• **90-Day mortality**: No significant difference
Secondary Outcome/s	• **SOFA Score at 6 hours, ICU LOS**: Significantly higher in EGDT group • **28-Day mortality, Hospital mortality, Hospital LOS, SOFA Score at 72 hours, Advanced organ support requirement**: No significant difference
Viva Summary	In a study comparing EGDT to standard care for patients with septic shock, there was no significant difference in 90-day mortality. However, the EGDT group had significantly higher SOFA scores at 6 hours and longer ICU LOS. Other secondary outcomes, including 28-day mortality, hospital mortality, hospital LOS, SOFA Score at 72 hours, and the requirement for advanced organ support, were not significantly different.
Study Conclusion	'In patients with septic shock who were identified early and received intravenous antibiotics and adequate fluid resuscitation, hemodynamic management according to a strict EGDT protocol did not lead to an improvement in outcome.'

ProMISe (2015): Mouncey PR, Osborn TM, Power S, et al. Trial of early, goal-directed resuscitation for septic shock. N Engl J Med. 2015;372(14): 1301–1311.

ACTIVATED PROTEIN C IN SEPSIS

Study Name	PROWESS (2001)
Population	Severe sepsis
Intervention	Drotrecogin alfa (activated) vs placebo
Primary Outcome/s	• **28-Day mortality**: Significantly lower in drotrecogin alfa group
Secondary Outcome/s	• **Incidence of serious bleeding**: Higher in the drotrecogin alfa group during the infusion period only • **Overall incidence of serious adverse events**: No significant difference
Viva Summary	In a study comparing drotrecogin alfa (activated) to a placebo for severe sepsis treatment, the drotrecogin alfa group had significantly lower 28-day mortality rates. However, there was a higher incidence of serious bleeding in the Drotrecogin alfa group, but only during the infusion period, with no significant difference in overall serious adverse events between the two groups.
Study Conclusion	'Treatment with drotrecogin alfa activated significantly reduces mortality in patients with severe sepsis and may be associated with an increased risk of bleeding.'

PROWESS (2001): Bernard GR, Vincent J, Laterre P, et al. Efficacy and safety of recombinant human activated protein C for severe sepsis. N Engl J Med. 2001;344(10):699–709.

Study Name	PROWESS-SHOCK (2012)
Population	Septic shock
Intervention	Drotrecogin alfa (activated) vs placebo
Primary Outcome/s	• **28-Day mortality**: No significant difference
Secondary Outcome/s	• **90-Day mortality, SOFA at day 7, Serious bleeding events**: No significant difference
Viva Summary	In a study comparing drotrecogin alfa (activated) to a placebo for treating septic shock, there was no significant difference in 28-day mortality or secondary outcomes including 90-day mortality, SOFA score at day 7, or serious bleeding events.
Study Conclusion	'Drotrecogin alfa (activated) did not significantly reduce mortality at 28 or 90 days, as compared with placebo, in patients with septic shock.'

PROWESS-SHOCK (2012): Ranieri VM, Thompson BT, Barie PS, et al. Drotrecogin alfa (activated) in adults with septic shock. N Engl J Med. 2012;366(22):2055–2064.

VITAMIN SUPPLEMENTATION IN SEPSIS

Study Name	Marik et al. (2017)
Population	Patients with severe sepsis or septic shock
Intervention	Treatment with IV vitamin C + hydrocortisone + thiamine vs standard care
Primary Outcome/s	• **Hospital mortality**: Significantly lower in treatment group
Secondary Outcome/s	• **Duration of vasopressors, Requirement for RRT**: Significantly lower in treatment group • **ICU LOS**: No significant difference • **Controversies**: Allegations of research fraud submitted in 2022
Viva Summary	In a study involving patients with severe sepsis or septic shock, treatment with IV vitamin C, hydrocortisone, and thiamine resulted in significantly lower hospital mortality. There was also a significant reduction in duration of vasopressor use and need for RRT compared to standard care. However, there was no significant difference in ICU LOS. In 2022, allegations of research fraud were raised regarding the study.
Study Conclusion	'Our results suggest that the early use of intravenous vitamin C, together with corticosteroids and thiamine, are effective in preventing progressive organ dysfunction, including acute kidney injury, and in reducing the mortality of patients with severe sepsis and septic shock. Additional studies are required to confirm these preliminary findings.'

Marik PE, Khangoora V, Rivera R, et al. Hydrocortisone, vitamin C, and thiamine for the treatment of severe sepsis and septic shock: a retrospective before-after study. Chest. 2017;151(6):1229–1238.

Study Name	CITRIS-ALI (2019)
Population	Patients with sepsis and ARDS
Intervention	IV vitamin C vs placebo
Primary Outcome/s	• **Change in modified SOFA Score, CRP, Thrombomodulin**: No significant difference
Secondary Outcome/s	Out of 46 prespecified secondary outcomes, 3 were significant: • **28-Day mortality**: Significantly lower in vitamin C group • **ICU-free days to day 28, Hospital-free days to day 60**: Significantly higher in vitamin C group
Viva Summary	In a study involving patients with sepsis and ARDS, the use of IV vitamin C compared to placebo did not show a significant difference in primary outcomes, including modified SOFA Score, CRP, and thrombomodulin. However, the vitamin C group had a significantly lower 28-day mortality and more ICU-free and hospital-free days up to day 28 and day 60, respectively.
Study Conclusion	'In this preliminary study of patients with sepsis and ARDS, a 96-hour infusion of vitamin C compared with placebo did not significantly improve organ dysfunction scores or alter markers of inflammation and vascular injury. Further research is needed to evaluate the potential role of vitamin C for other outcomes in sepsis and ARDS.'

CITRIS-ALI (2019): Fowler AA, Truwit JD, Hite RD, et al. Effect of vitamin C infusion on organ failure and biomarkers of inflammation and vascular injury in patients with sepsis and severe acute respiratory failure: the CITRIS-ALI randomized clinical trial. JAMA 2019;322(13):1261–1270.

Study Name	VITAMINS (2020)
Population	Patients with septic shock meeting the Sepsis-3 definition
Intervention	Vitamin C + hydrocortisone + thiamine vs hydrocortisone alone until shock resolution or up to 10 days
Primary Outcome/s	• **Duration of time alive and free of vasopressor administration up to day 7**: No significant difference
Secondary Outcome/s	• **SOFA Score at day 3**: Significantly greater improvement in intervention group • Nine other prespecified secondary outcomes showed no statistically significant difference
Viva Summary	In a study involving patients with septic shock, the group receiving vitamin C, hydrocortisone, and thiamine did not have a significantly different duration of time without vasopressor administration up to day 7 compared to the group receiving hydrocortisone alone. However, the intervention group did experience a significantly greater improvement in SOFA Score at day 3, while other pre-specified secondary outcomes did not exhibit statistically significant differences.
Study Conclusion	'In patients with septic shock, treatment with intravenous vitamin C, hydrocortisone, and thiamine, compared with intravenous hydrocortisone alone, did not significantly improve the duration of time alive and free of vasopressor administration over 7 days. The finding suggests that treatment with intravenous vitamin C, hydrocortisone, and thiamine does not lead to a more rapid resolution of septic shock compared with intravenous hydrocortisone alone.'

VITAMINS (2020): Fujii T, Luethi N, Young PJ, Frei DR et al.; VITAMINS Trial Investigators. Effect of vitamin C, hydrocortisone, and thiamine vs hydrocortisone alone on time alive and free of vasopressor support among patients with septic shock: the VITAMINS randomized clinical trial. JAMA. 2020 Feb 4;323(5):423–431.

Study Name	VICTAS (2021)
Population	Adult patients with sepsis-induced respiratory and/or cardiovascular dysfunction
Intervention	Vitamin C + hydrocortisone + thiamine vs placebo
Primary Outcome/s	• **Number of consecutive ventilator- and vasopressor-free days in the first 30 days**: No significant difference
Secondary Outcome/s	• **30-Day mortality**: No significant difference
Viva Summary	In a study involving adult patients with sepsis-induced respiratory and cardiovascular dysfunction, the use of vitamin C, hydrocortisone, and thiamine did not show a significant difference in the number of consecutive ventilator- and vasopressor-free days in the first 30 days or in 30-day mortality when compared to a placebo.
Study conclusion	'Among critically ill patients with sepsis, treatment with vitamin C, thiamine, and hydrocortisone, compared with placebo, did not significantly increase ventilator- and vasopressor-free days within 30 days. However, the trial was terminated early for administrative reasons and may have been underpowered to detect a clinically important difference.'

VICTAS (2021): Sevransky JE, Rothman RE, Hager DN, Bernard GR et al.; VICTAS Investigators. Effect of vitamin C, thiamine, and hydrocortisone on ventilator- and vasopressor-free days in patients with sepsis: the VICTAS randomized clinical trial. JAMA. 2021 Feb 23;325(8):742–750.

Study Name	LOVIT (2022)
Population	Sepsis requiring vasopressors
Intervention	High-dose vitamin C vs placebo
Primary Outcome/s	• **Composite of 28-day mortality or persistent organ dysfunction**: Significantly higher in vitamin C group
Secondary Outcome/s	• **Days without organ dysfunction, 6-month mortality, Quality of life, SOFA Score, Markers of tissue dysoxia (lactate), inflammation, and endothelial injury**: No significant difference
Viva Summary	In a study involving sepsis patients requiring vasopressors, high-dose vitamin C was compared to placebo. The primary outcome, a composite of 28-day mortality or persistent organ dysfunction, was significantly higher in the vitamin C group. However, there were no significant differences observed in secondary outcomes, including days without organ dysfunction, 6-month mortality, quality of life, SOFA Score or markers of tissue dysoxia, inflammation, and endothelial injury.
Study Conclusion	'In adults with sepsis receiving vasopressor therapy in the ICU, those who received intravenous vitamin C had a higher risk of death or persistent organ dysfunction at 28 days than those who received placebo.'

LOVIT (2022): Lamontagne F, Masse MH, Menard J, et al. Intravenous vitamin C in adults with sepsis in the intensive care unit. N Engl J Med. 2022;386(25):2387–2398.

CORTICOSTEROIDS IN SEPSIS

Study Name	CORTICUS (2008)
Population	Patients with septic shock
Intervention	Hydrocortisone 50 mg every 6 hours (tapering regimen from day 6, stopped on day 12) vs placebo
Primary Outcome/s	• **28-Day mortality in short corticotropin non-responders (i.e. the subgroup that was more likely to benefit from exogenous corticosteroids)**: No significant difference
Secondary Outcome/s	• **28-Day mortality in short corticotropin responders (i.e. the subgroup that was less likely to benefit from exogenous corticosteroids), 28-Day mortality in all patients**: No significant difference • **Time to reversal of shock**: Significantly shorter with hydrocortisone • **Rate of superinfections**: Non-significant increase
Viva Summary	In a study involving patients with septic shock, the administration of hydrocortisone 50 mg every 6 hours did not significantly impact 28-day mortality in either short corticotropin non-responders or responders. However, it did lead to a significantly shorter time to shock reversal.
Study Conclusion	'Hydrocortisone did not improve survival or reversal of shock in patients with septic shock, either overall or in patients who did not have a response to corticotropin, although hydrocortisone hastened reversal of shock in patients in whom shock was reversed.'

CORTICUS (2008): Sprung CL, Annane D, Keh D, et al. Hydrocortisone therapy for patients with septic shock. N Engl J Med. 2008;358(2):111–124.

Study Name	HYPRESS (2016)
Population	Adults with severe sepsis not in septic shock
Intervention	Continuous infusion of hydrocortisone 200 mg for 5 days followed by tapering until day 11 vs placebo
Primary Outcome/s	• **Development of septic shock within 14 days**: No significant difference
Secondary Outcome/s	• Secondary outcomes including time to septic shock or death, ICU and hospital mortality, vital status at various time points, ICU/hospital LOS, SOFA Score, duration of mechanical ventilation, and RRT did not differ significantly between groups • The hydrocortisone group had more episodes of hyperglycaemia but a lower incidence of delirium
Viva Summary	In a study involving adults with severe sepsis but not in septic shock, the continuous infusion of hydrocortisone at 200 mg for 5 days followed by tapering until day 11 did not significantly reduce the development of septic shock within 14 days when compared to a placebo. Secondary outcomes, including various measures of mortality, LOS, and complications, were not significantly different between the two groups. However, the hydrocortisone group did experience more episodes of hyperglycaemia but a lower incidence of delirium.
Study Conclusion	'Among adults with severe sepsis not in septic shock, use of hydrocortisone compared with placebo did not reduce the risk of septic shock within 14 days. These findings do not support the use of hydrocortisone in these patients.'

HYPRESS (2016): Keh D, Trips E, Marx G, Wirtz SP et al.; SepNet–Critical Care Trials Group. Effect of hydrocortisone on development of shock among patients with severe sepsis: the HYPRESS randomized clinical trial. JAMA. 2016 Nov 1;316(17):1775–1785.

Study Name	ADRENAL (2018)
Population	Patients with septic shock requiring vasopressors and mechanical ventilation
Intervention	• Hydrocortisone 200 mg/day IV infusion for 7 days or until ICU discharge vs placebo
Primary Outcome/s	• **90-Day mortality**: No significant difference
Secondary Outcome/s	• **Time to resolution of shock, Time to cessation of mechanical ventilation, Time to discharge from ICU, Use of blood transfusion**: Significantly lower in hydrocortisone group • **28-Day mortality, Recurrence of shock, Days alive and outside of the ICU, Days to hospital discharge, Days alive and outside of the hospital, Days alive and free of mechanical ventilation, Use of RRT**: No significant difference
Viva Summary	In a study involving patients with septic shock needing vasopressors and mechanical ventilation, the administration of hydrocortisone 200 mg/day IV infusion for 7 days or until ICU discharge did not significantly affect 90-day mortality compared to placebo. However, the hydrocortisone group had significant reductions in various secondary outcomes, including time to resolution of shock, time to cessation of mechanical ventilation, time to discharge from ICU, and use of blood transfusion.
Study Conclusion	'Among patients with septic shock undergoing mechanical ventilation, a continuous infusion of hydrocortisone did not result in lower 90-day mortality than placebo.'

ADRENAL (2018): Venkatesh B, Finfer S, Cohen J, et al. Adjunctive glucocorticoid therapy in patients with septic shock. N Engl J Med. 2018;378(9): 797–808.

Study Name	APROCCHSS (2018)
Population	Patients with septic shock requiring vasopressors
Intervention	IV hydrocortisone 50 mg 6 hourly + oral fludrocortisone 50 µg daily for 7 days vs placebo
Primary Outcome/s	• **90-Day mortality**: Significantly lower in the intervention group
Secondary Outcome/s	• **All-cause mortality at ICU/hospital discharge and at 180 days**: Significantly lower in the intervention group • **Days free from vasopressors, Organ-failure-free days**: Significantly more in the intervention group • **Serious adverse events**: No significant difference
Viva Summary	In a study involving patients with septic shock requiring vasopressors, the intervention group received IV hydrocortisone and oral fludrocortisone for 7 days, while the placebo group did not. The primary outcome of 90-day mortality was significantly lower in the intervention group. Additionally, secondary outcomes, including all-cause mortality at ICU/hospital discharge and at 180 days, days free from vasopressors, and organ failure-free days, were significantly more favourable in the intervention group. There was no significant difference in serious adverse events between the two groups.
Study Conclusion	'In this trial involving patients with septic shock, 90-day all-cause mortality was lower among those who received hydrocortisone plus fludrocortisone than among those who received placebo.'

APROCCHSS (2018): Annane D, Renault A, Brun-Buisson C, et al. Hydrocortisone plus fludrocortisone for adults with septic shock. N Engl J Med. 2018;378(9):809–818.

BETA-BLOCKERS IN SEPSIS

Study Name	STRESS-L (2023)
Population	Adults in ICU with septic shock, HR ≥95 bpm, on >0.1 mcg/kg/min norepinephrine for 24–72 hours
Intervention	Landiolol infusion (started at 1 mcg/kg/min, titrated to achieve HR of 80–94 bpm) vs standard care (no beta-blockade)
Primary Outcome/s	• **Mean SOFA Score over first 14 days**: No significant difference
Secondary Outcome/s	• **28-Day mortality, 90-Day mortality, ICU/Hospital LOS, Mean lactate/PaO_2/$PaCO_2$**: No significant difference • **Average norepinephrine infusion rate, Serious adverse events**: Significantly higher in landiolol group • **Heart rate over 14 days**: Significantly lower in landiolol group
Viva Summary	In a study involving adults in ICU with septic shock and HR ≥95 bpm on norepinephrine for 24–72 hours, the effects of a landiolol infusion (target HR 80–94 bpm) were compared to standard care (no beta-blockade). The primary outcome, mean SOFA Score over the first 14 days, was not significantly different. Additionally, secondary outcomes, including 28-day mortality, 90-day mortality, ICU/hospital LOS, and mean lactate/PaO_2/$PaCO_2$ levels, were not significantly different. However, the landiolol group had a significantly higher average norepinephrine infusion rate and experienced more serious adverse events.
Study Conclusion	'Among patients with septic shock with tachycardia and treated with norepinephrine for more than 24 hours, an infusion of landiolol did not reduce organ failure measured by the SOFA score over 14 days from randomization. These results do not support the use of landiolol for managing tachycardia among patients treated with norepinephrine for established septic shock.'

STRESS-L (2023): Whitehouse T, Hossain A, Perkins GD, et al. Landiolol and organ failure in patients with septic shock: the STRESS-L randomized clinical trial. JAMA. 2023;330(17):1641–1652.

SUMMARY

1. **SAFE (2004):** In a study comparing resuscitation with 4% HAS to 0.9% NaCl, there was no significant difference in 28-day all-cause mortality, LOS, duration of mechanical ventilation, or RRT duration. However, post-hoc analysis revealed a significantly higher 28-day mortality in TBI patients who received 4% HAS.

2. **FEAST (2011):** In a resource-limited African setting, a study compared the use of fluid bolus (5% HAS or 0.9% saline) to no fluid bolus in paediatric patients with severe febrile illness. The study found that 48-hour mortality was significantly higher in the fluid bolus group for patients without severe hypotension, and the overall 4-week mortality was also significantly higher in the fluid bolus group.

3. **CHEST (2012):** In a study comparing the use of 6% HES to 0.9% NaCl for fluid resuscitation in critically ill patients, there was no significant difference in 90-day mortality between the two groups. However, the HES group experienced significantly higher rates of renal impairment, use of RRT, and adverse events, while there was no significant difference in the duration of mechanical ventilation or duration of RRT.

4. **SPLIT (2015):** In a study comparing Plasma-Lyte 148 and 0.9% NaCl for ICU patients requiring crystalloid fluid therapy, there was no significant difference in the proportion of patients developing AKI within 90 days or in secondary outcomes such as AKI incidence, need for RRT, ICU readmission, LOS, or mortality rates.

5. **SMART (2018):** In a study comparing balanced crystalloids to 0.9% NaCl for critically ill patients, the primary outcome of Major Adverse Kidney Events (MAKEs) at 30 days was significantly lower with balanced crystalloids. However, there were no significant differences in secondary outcomes such as mortality, new need for RRT, persistent renal dysfunction, VFDs, or vasopressor-free days.

6. **BaSICS (2021):** In a study comparing Plasma-Lyte and 0.9% NaCl for adult ICU patients, administered via slow or rapid bolus, there was no significant difference in 90-day mortality. However, the secondary outcome of day 7 SOFA Score was significantly lower

with Plasma-Lyte, while the other secondary outcomes, including AKI requiring RRT within 90 days, were not significantly different between the intervention groups.

7. **PLUS (2022):** In a study comparing Plasma-Lyte and 0.9% NaCl for adult ICU patients, there was no significant difference in 90-day mortality or secondary outcomes such as need for RRT, days free of mechanical ventilation, use of vasoactive drugs, or serum creatinine levels.

8. **PREPARE II (2022):** In a study involving critically ill adult patients requiring tracheal intubation and positive pressure ventilation, the administration of a 500-ml fluid bolus showed no significant difference in the incidence of cardiovascular collapse or in-hospital mortality at 28 days compared to not receiving a fluid bolus.

9. **PAC-Man (2005):** In a study comparing the use of PAC to no PAC in critically ill patients, there was no significant difference in hospital mortality or secondary outcomes such as ICU/hospital LOS or organ support. However, the PAC group experienced a 10% complication rate, including haematoma, arterial puncture, arrhythmia, PTX, HTX, and lost guidewire.

10. **CRASH-2 (2010):** In a study involving trauma patients with/at risk of significant haemorrhage, the early administration of TXA significantly reduced hospital mortality within 4 weeks of injury compared to placebo. However, there was no significant difference in transfusion requirements, vaso-occlusive events, or dependency between the two groups.

11. **PROPPR (2015):** In a study comparing a 1:1:1 ratio of plasma:platelets:red cells to a 1:1:2 ratio for severe trauma patients requiring massive transfusion, there were no significant differences in 24-hour and 30-day mortality rates. There were also no differences in various secondary outcomes including complications, time to achieve haemostasis, or functional status at discharge. However, a post-hoc analysis did reveal a significant reduction in death due to exsanguination within the first 24 hours and a higher rate of achieving haemostasis in the 1:1:1 ratio group compared to the 1:1:2 ratio group.

12. **CRYOSTAT-1 (2015):** In a study on trauma patients, the addition of two early pools of cryoprecipitate to standard care was found to be feasible, with 85% of subjects in the intervention arm receiving cryoprecipitate within 90 minutes. There was no significant difference in 28-day all-cause mortality between the intervention and standard care groups, but the intervention group had higher fibrinogen concentrations.

13. **ITACTIC (2020):** In a study comparing the use of viscoelastic haemostatic assays (VHA) to conventional coagulation tests (CCT) in managing major haemorrhage with shock, there was no significant difference in the primary outcome of survival without massive transfusion at 24 hours. Additionally, no significant differences were observed in any secondary outcomes overall. However, in a sub-group analysis of patients with severe TBI, the VHA group showed a significantly lower 28-day mortality rate compared to the CCT group.

14. **PATCH (2023):** In a study involving adult trauma patients at risk for trauma-induced coagulopathy (COAST score >3), early administration of 1g TXA followed by an 8-hour TXA infusion did not significantly affect survival with favourable functional outcomes at 6 months. However, the TXA group showed significantly reduced mortality at 24 hours and 28 days, and post-hoc analysis suggested better neurological outcomes for patients with an AIS ≤2 in the head or neck region. Other secondary outcomes, such as 6-month mortality and various coagulation measures, did not differ significantly between the two groups.

15. **PARAMEDIC2 (2018):** In a study comparing adrenaline to placebo for OHCA, the adrenaline group had significantly higher 30-day survival rates but also a significantly higher incidence of severe neurological impairment (mRS 4–5). There was no significant difference in survival with favourable outcomes or ICU/hospital LOS between the two groups.

16. **ARREST (2020):** In a study comparing early ECMO to conventional resuscitation for OHCA patients with initial rhythm of VF or pulseless VT, the early ECMO group showed significantly higher survival rates both at hospital discharge and at the 6-month mark. The study was stopped early due to strong evidence favouring ECMO, with a posterior probability of 0.9861 exceeding the predetermined threshold of 0.986.

17. **TOMAHAWK (2021):** In a study of OHCA patients aged over 30 without ST-segment elevation, immediate angiography did not significantly change 30-day mortality compared to delayed/selective angiography. However, the immediate angiography group had a notably higher rate of a composite outcome involving 30-day mortality or severe neurological deficit. Other factors such as peak troponin release, bleeding, stroke, and RRT incidence exhibited no significant differences between the two groups.

18. **BOX (Blood Pressure) (2022):** In a study involving comatose survivors of an OHCA, there was no significant difference in death or hospital discharge with a Cerebral Performance Score of 3–4 between those treated with a higher MAP target (>77 mmHg) and those with a standard MAP target (>63 mmHg) up to day 90. Additionally, there were no significant differences in secondary outcomes, including 90-day mortality, neuron-specific enolase levels, and adverse event rates.

19. **INCEPTION (2023):** In a study involving patients with refractory OHCA and an initial ventricular arrhythmia, the use of ECPR did not significantly improve survival with a favourable neurological outcome at 30 days compared to conventional CPR. Additionally, the ECPR group had a higher rate of admission to ICU, with no significant differences in 3-month or 6-month survival with a favourable neurological outcome.

20. **IMPROVE (2014):** In a study comparing EVAR to open repair for ruptured AAA, there was no significant difference in 30-day mortality rate between the two interventions. However, EVAR with local anaesthesia alone resulted in a four-fold reduction in 30-day mortality compared to general anaesthesia. Additionally, maintaining permissive hypotension with an SBP <70 mmHg was independently associated with a high 30-day mortality rate of 51%.

21. **ISIS-2 (1988):** In a study comparing treatments for acute MI with a 24-hour symptom onset, streptokinase alone reduced vascular mortality by 25%, aspirin alone reduced it by 23%, and the combination of both reduced it by 40% at 5 weeks. Combining streptokinase and aspirin also lowered reinfarction, stroke, and death rates compared to no treatment, and these benefits remained significant after 15 months of follow-up.

22. **NORDISTEMI (2010):** In a study comparing immediate PCI to PCI for rescue/deterioration in STEMI patients post-thrombolysis, the primary composite outcome of death, reinfarction, stroke, or new ischaemia at 1 year was not significantly different between the treatment groups. However, the secondary composite outcome of death, reinfarction, or stroke at 12 months was significantly lower in the immediate PCI group. Bleeding and infarct size were not significantly different.

23. **POISE (2008):** In a study involving patients undergoing non-cardiac surgery, those who received metoprolol succinate before and after the operation had a significantly lower rate of a composite outcome, which included cardiovascular death, non-fatal MI, and non-fatal cardiac arrest at 30 days, compared to those who received a placebo. They also had significantly lower rates of new clinically significant atrial fibrillation and the need for cardiac revascularisation. However, the metoprolol group also had significantly higher 30-day all-cause mortality, stroke, clinically significant hypotension, and bradycardia.

24. **SHOCK (1999):** In a study comparing emergency revascularisation (CABG/angioplasty) to initial medical stabilisation for patients with shock due to LV failure following an MI, there was no significant difference in 30-day mortality. However, the emergency revascularisation group had a significantly lower 6-month mortality rate.

25. **REMATCH (2001):** In a study comparing LVAD intervention to medical management for end-stage heart failure, the LVAD group had significantly lower all-cause mortality at 1 and 2 years and improved quality of life. However, the LVAD group also experienced significantly more serious adverse events, mainly related to infection, bleeding, and device malfunction.

26. **IABP-SHOCK II (2012):** In a study comparing the use of an IABP to medical therapy for patients with an acute MI and cardiogenic shock, there was no significant difference in 30-day all-cause mortality or secondary outcomes including reinfarction, peripheral ischaemia, bleeding, or sepsis.

27. **ECMO-CS (2022):** In a study comparing the use of immediate VA-ECMO versus conservative therapy in patients with severe cardiogenic shock, there was no significant difference in the

composite outcome of death, resuscitated cardiac arrest, or the need for another mechanical circulatory support at 30 days. Additionally, no significant differences were observed in secondary outcomes or serious adverse events.

28. **MIDAS (2020):** In a study comparing 20 mg of midodrine administered every 8 hours to a placebo in adults on single-agent vasopressors, no significant difference was found in the overall time to vasopressor discontinuation. However, a post-hoc analysis showed a significant reduction in discontinuation time among patients with epidural analgesia. Secondary outcomes, including readiness for ICU discharge, ICU/hospital LOS, and ICU readmission rates, showed no significant differences. Notably, bradycardia rates were significantly higher in the midodrine group.

29. **6S (2012):** In a study comparing the use of 6% HES to Ringer's acetate in critically ill adults with severe sepsis, the HES group had significantly higher rates of death or dialysis dependence at 90 days, as well as a significantly higher use of RRT compared to the Ringer's acetate group.

30. **ALBIOS (2014):** In a study involving adults with severe sepsis or septic shock, administering 20% HAS along with crystalloid to maintain a target serum albumin level of ≥30 g/l did not lead to a significant difference in 28-day or 90-day mortality when compared to the use of crystalloid alone.

31. **CLASSIC (2022):** In a study involving adult ICU patients with septic shock, a comparison was made between restrictive fluid therapy and standard care. The primary outcome of 90-day mortality was not significantly different between the two groups. Similarly, secondary outcomes, including serious adverse events, days alive without life support, and days alive and out of the hospital, were not significantly different.

32. **VASST (2008):** In a study comparing vasopressin at 0.01–0.03 units/min to norepinephrine at 5–15 μg/min for septic shock, there was no significant difference in 28-day mortality or various secondary outcomes, including 90-day mortality, need for RRT, LOS, organ dysfunction, and adverse events. However, the vasopressin group did have a significantly lower norepinephrine infusion rate, and a post-hoc analysis suggested a potential advantage of vasopressin in patients with less severe shock.

33. **SOAP II (2010):** In a study comparing the use of dopamine and noradrenaline in patients with circulatory shock, there was no significant difference in 28-day mortality. However, dopamine was associated with fewer vasopressor-free days, higher rates of death from refractory shock, increased arrhythmias, and higher 28-day mortality in cardiogenic shock. There were no significant differences in days without ICU care or days without organ support.

34. **VANISH (2016):** In a study involving adult patients with septic shock requiring vasopressors despite fluid resuscitation, four treatment groups were compared: 1) vasopressin + hydrocortisone, 2) vasopressin + placebo, 3) noradrenaline + hydrocortisone, and 4) noradrenaline + placebo. The primary outcome of kidney failure-free days during the 28-day period was not significantly different between the groups. Analysis of secondary outcomes revealed no significant differences in outcomes such as mortality rates, kidney failure rates, or SOFA scores, but did show lower rates of RRT in the vasopressin groups.

35. **LeoPARDS (2016):** In a study comparing levosimendan to a placebo for adults with sepsis, there was no difference in mean daily SOFA Score up to day 28. However, the levosimendan group had a lower likelihood of successful weaning from mechanical ventilation over 28 days and a higher risk of supraventricular tachyarrhythmias. There was no significant difference in 28-day mortality.

36. **CLOVERS (2023):** In a study involving adult sepsis patients with hypotension, a comparison was made between a restrictive fluid strategy with early vasopressor use and a liberal fluid strategy with later vasopressor use. The primary outcome of all-cause mortality before discharge was not significantly different between the two strategies at 90 days. Additionally, there were no significant differences in secondary outcomes, except for a higher rate of ICU admissions in the restrictive fluid group during the initial 7 days on post-hoc analysis.

37. **TRISS (2014):** In a study involving patients with septic shock, two transfusion thresholds were compared: ≤70 g/l (lower) and ≤90 g/l (higher). There was no significant difference in 90-day mortality between the groups. However, the lower threshold group required significantly fewer transfusions and a higher proportion of patients did not undergo any transfusion at all compared to the higher threshold group.

38. **SEPSISPAM (2014):** In a study involving patients with septic shock, a comparison was made between two MAP targets: a higher target of 80–85 mmHg and a lower target of 65–70 mmHg. There was no difference in 28-day mortality between the two groups. Similarly, there were no significant differences in 90-day mortality or serious adverse events. However, the 80–85 mmHg target group had a significantly higher rate of new AF. Subgroup analysis in patients with chronic hypertension revealed that the high MAP group required RRT less frequently from day 1 to 7 compared to the lower MAP group.

39. **ANDROMEDA-SHOCK (2019):** In a study involving patients with septic shock, there was no significant difference in 28-day mortality between those receiving resuscitation to normalise capillary refill time and those aiming to decrease lactate levels over an 8-hour period. However, the group focused on capillary refill time normalisation exhibited significantly lower organ dysfunction at 72 hours. Secondary outcomes such as 90-day mortality, organ support-free days, and LOS were not significantly different between the two intervention groups.

40. **65 (2020):** In a study involving patients over 65 years with vasodilatory hypotension who were initiated on vasopressors, a comparison was made between permissive hypotension (targeting a MAP of 60–65 mmHg) and standard care. Ninety-day mortality was not significantly different between the two groups; however, the permissive hypotension group had significantly lower exposure to vasopressors. Other secondary outcomes, such as ICU/hospital mortality, duration of organ support, LOS, cognitive decline, and quality of life, were not significantly different. Subgroup analysis suggested potential survival benefits for chronically hypertensive patients in the permissive hypotension group and a possible trend towards improved survival with increasing age.

41. **Rivers et al. (2001):** In a study involving patients with severe sepsis or septic shock, EGDT was compared to standard care. The results showed that EGDT led to significantly lower in-hospital mortality, reduced severity of sepsis, and lower mortality rates at 28 and 60 days.

42. **ARISE (2014):** In a study comparing EGDT to standard care for patients with septic shock, there was no significant difference in 90-day all-cause mortality. However, the use of vasopressors and red cell transfusions was significantly higher in the EGDT group.

Other secondary outcomes, including ED/hospital LOS, duration of time on vasopressors, RRT, and mechanical ventilation, were not significantly different between the two groups.

43. **ProCESS (2014):** In a study comparing the treatment of patients with sepsis, three interventions were examined: 6 hours of EGDT, protocol-guided standard care, and usual care. The primary outcome, 60-day mortality, was not significantly different between the three groups. Similarly, there were no significant differences in secondary outcomes including 90-day mortality and 1-year mortality.

44. **ProMISe (2015):** In a study comparing EGDT to standard care for patients with septic shock, there was no significant difference in 90-day mortality. However, the EGDT group had significantly higher SOFA scores at 6 hours and longer ICU LOS. Other secondary outcomes, including 28-day mortality, hospital mortality, hospital LOS, SOFA Score at 72 hours, and the requirement for advanced organ support, were not significantly different.

45. **PROWESS (2001):** In a study comparing drotrecogin alfa (activated) to a placebo for severe sepsis treatment, the drotrecogin alfa group had significantly lower 28-day mortality rates. However, there was a higher incidence of serious bleeding in the drotrecogin alfa group, but only during the infusion period, with no significant difference in overall serious adverse events between the two groups.

46. **PROWESS-SHOCK (2012):** In a study comparing drotrecogin alfa (activated) to a placebo for treating septic shock, there was no significant difference in 28-day mortality or secondary outcomes including 90-day mortality, SOFA Score at day 7, or serious bleeding events.

47. **Marik et al. (2017):** In a study involving patients with severe sepsis or septic shock, treatment with IV vitamin C, hydrocortisone, and thiamine resulted in significantly lower hospital mortality. There was also a significant reduction in duration of vasopressor use and need for RRT compared to standard care. However, there was no significant difference in ICU LOS. In 2022, allegations of research fraud were raised regarding the study.

48. **CITRIS-ALI (2019):** In a study involving patients with sepsis and ARDS, the use of IV vitamin C compared to placebo did not show a significant difference in primary outcomes, including modified

SOFA Score, CRP, and thrombomodulin. However, the vitamin C group had a significantly lower 28-day mortality and more ICU-free and hospital-free days up to day 28 and day 60, respectively.

49. **VITAMINS (2020):** In a study involving patients with septic shock, the group receiving vitamin C, hydrocortisone, and thiamine did not have a significantly different duration of time without vasopressor administration up to day 7 compared to the group receiving hydrocortisone alone. However, the intervention group did experience a significantly greater improvement in SOFA Score at day 3, while other prespecified secondary outcomes did not exhibit statistically significant differences.

50. **VICTAS (2021):** In a study involving adult patients with sepsis-induced respiratory and cardiovascular dysfunction, the use of vitamin C, hydrocortisone, and thiamine did not show a significant difference in the number of consecutive ventilator- and vasopressor-free days in the first 30 days or in 30-day mortality when compared to a placebo.

51. **LOVIT (2022):** In a study involving sepsis patients requiring vasopressors, high-dose vitamin C was compared to placebo. The primary outcome, a composite of 28-day mortality or persistent organ dysfunction, was significantly higher in the vitamin C group. However, there were no significant differences observed in secondary outcomes, including days without organ dysfunction, 6-month mortality, quality of life, SOFA Score or markers of tissue dysoxia, inflammation, and endothelial injury.

52. **CORTICUS (2008):** In a study involving patients with septic shock, the administration of hydrocortisone 50 mg every 6 hours did not significantly impact 28-day mortality in either short corticotropin non-responders or responders. However, it did lead to a significantly shorter time to shock reversal.

53. **HYPRESS (2016):** In a study involving adults with severe sepsis but not in septic shock, the continuous infusion of hydrocortisone at 200 mg for 5 days followed by tapering until day 11 did not significantly reduce the development of septic shock within 14 days when compared to a placebo. Secondary outcomes, including various measures of mortality, LOS, and complications, were not significantly different between the two groups. However, the hydrocortisone group did experience more episodes of hyperglycaemia but a lower incidence of delirium.

54. **ADRENAL (2018):** In a study involving patients with septic shock needing vasopressors and mechanical ventilation, the administration of hydrocortisone 200 mg/day IV infusion for 7 days or until ICU discharge did not significantly affect 90-day mortality compared to placebo. However, the hydrocortisone group had significant reductions in various secondary outcomes, including time to resolution of shock, time to cessation of mechanical ventilation, time to discharge from ICU, and use of blood transfusion.

55. **APROCCHSS (2018):** In a study involving patients with septic shock requiring vasopressors, the intervention group received IV hydrocortisone and oral fludrocortisone for 7 days, while the placebo group did not. The primary outcome of 90-day mortality was significantly lower in the intervention group. Additionally, secondary outcomes, including all-cause mortality at ICU/hospital discharge and at 180 days, days free from vasopressors, and organ failure–free days, were significantly more favourable in the intervention group. There was no significant difference in serious adverse events between the two groups.

56. **STRESS-L (2023):** In a study involving adults in ICU with septic shock and HR ≥95 bpm on norepinephrine for 24–72 hours, the effects of a landiolol infusion (target HR 80–94 bpm) were compared to standard care (no beta-blockade). The primary outcome, mean SOFA Score over the first 14 days, was not significantly different. Additionally, secondary outcomes, including 28-day mortality, 90-day mortality, ICU/hospital LOS, and mean lactate/ $PaO_2/PaCO_2$ levels, were not significantly different. However, the landiolol group had a significantly higher average norepinephrine infusion rate and experienced more serious adverse events.

CHAPTER 3
NEUROLOGY AND SEDATION

SEDATION

Study Name	ABC (2008)
Population	Mechanically ventilated and sedated patients
Intervention	Spontaneous awakening trial (SAT) followed by spontaneous breathing trial (SBT) vs SBT alone (control group)
Primary Outcome/s	• **VFDs to day 28**: Significantly higher in the intervention group
Secondary Outcome/s	• **ICU/Hospital LOS, 1-Year mortality**: Significantly lower in intervention group • **Self-extubation**: Significantly higher in intervention group • **Reintubation rates**: No significant difference (even after self-extubation)
Viva Summary	In a study involving mechanically ventilated and sedated patients, the intervention group underwent an SAT followed by an SBT, while the control group received an SBT alone. The intervention group had significantly more VFDs by day 28, lower ICU/hospital LOS, and lower 1-year mortality. However, the intervention group also had a higher rate of self-extubation, with no significant difference in reintubation rates, even after self-extubation.
Study Conclusion	'Our results suggest that a wake up and breathe protocol that pairs daily spontaneous awakening trials (ie, interruption of sedatives) with daily spontaneous breathing trials results in better outcomes for mechanically ventilated patients in intensive care than current standard approaches and should become routine practice.'

ABC (2008): Girard TD, Kress JP, Fuchs BD, et al. Efficacy and safety of a paired sedation and ventilator weaning protocol for mechanically ventilated patients in intensive care (Awakening and Breathing Controlled trial): a randomised controlled trial. Lancet. 2008;371(9607):126–134.

DOI: 10.1201/9781003468738-3

Study Name	SLEAP (2012)
Population	Mechanically ventilated patients sedated with opioids and/or benzodiazepines
Intervention	Daily sedation interruption vs no planned sedation interruption
Primary Outcome/s	• **Days to extubation**: No significant difference
Secondary Outcome/s	• **Doses of sedatives/analgesics, Nurse/respiratory therapist clinical workload**: Higher in interruption group • **Days to extubation in trauma and surgical patients**: Significantly lower in interruption group (subgroup analysis) • **ICU LOS, Rates of delirium, Unintentional device removal**: No significant difference
Viva Summary	In a study involving mechanically ventilated patients sedated with opioids and/or benzodiazepines, the primary outcome of days to extubation was not significantly different between the group receiving daily sedation interruption and the group with no planned sedation interruption. However, in a subgroup analysis of trauma and surgical patients, the interruption group experienced significantly fewer days to extubation. Additionally, the interruption group required higher doses of sedatives/analgesics and resulted in a higher nurse/respiratory therapist clinical workload. There were no significant differences in ICU LOS, rates of delirium, or unintentional device removal between the two groups.
Study Conclusion	'For mechanically ventilated adults managed with protocolized sedation, the addition of daily sedation interruption did not reduce the duration of mechanical ventilation or ICU stay.'

SLEAP (2012): Mehta S, Burry L, Cook D, et al. Daily sedation interruption in mechanically ventilated critically ill patients cared for with a sedation protocol: a randomized controlled trial. JAMA. 2012;308(19):1985–1992.

Study Name	MIDEX-PRODEX (2012)
Population	Adult ICU patients receiving prolonged mechanical ventilation
Intervention	• MIDEX trial: Sedation with dexmedetomidine vs midazolam • PRODEX trial: Sedation with dexmedetomidine vs propofol
Primary Outcome/s	• **Maintaining target sedation level**: Dexmedetomidine was non-inferior to midazolam and propofol • **Duration of mechanical ventilation**: Significantly shorter for dexmedetomidine compared with midazolam, but **not** for dexmedetomidine compared with propofol
Secondary Outcome/s	• **Median time to extubation**: Significantly shorter for dexmedetomidine compared with midazolam and propofol • **Ability to communicate pain, arousability, and cooperation of the patient**: Significantly higher with dexmedetomidine compared with midazolam and propofol • **Incidence of hypotension and bradycardia**: Significantly higher with dexmedetomidine compared to midazolam • **ICU LOS**: No significant difference
Viva Summary	Two trials, MIDEX and PRODEX, compared dexmedetomidine with midazolam and propofol in adult ICU patients on prolonged mechanical ventilation. Dexmedetomidine was found to be non-inferior to both midazolam and propofol in maintaining target sedation levels. However, the duration of mechanical ventilation was significantly shorter with dexmedetomidine compared to midazolam, but not propofol. Dexmedetomidine also led to a significantly shorter median time to extubation and improved patient outcomes in terms of pain communication, arousability, and cooperation, compared to both alternatives. However, it was associated with a higher incidence of hypotension and bradycardia than midazolam. There was no significant difference in ICU LOS between the groups.

(Continued)

(Continued)

Study Name	MIDEX-PRODEX (2012)
Study Conclusion	'Among ICU patients receiving prolonged mechanical ventilation, dexmedetomidine was not inferior to midazolam and propofol in maintaining light to moderate sedation. Dexmedetomidine reduced duration of mechanical ventilation compared with midazolam and improved patients' ability to communicate pain compared with midazolam and propofol. More adverse effects were associated with dexmedetomidine.'

MIDEX-PRODEX Trial (2012): Jakob SM, Ruokonen E, Grounds RM, Sarapohja T et al.; Dexmedetomidine for Long-Term Sedation Investigators. Dexmedetomidine vs midazolam or propofol for sedation during prolonged mechanical ventilation: two randomized controlled trials. JAMA. 2012 Mar 21;307(11):1151–1160.

THERAPEUTIC HYPOTHERMIA POST-OHCA

Study Name	TTM (2013)
Population	Unconscious patients after OHCA (of presumed cardiac cause)
Intervention	Targeted temperature management (TTM) of 33°C vs 36°C
Primary Outcome/s	• **All-cause mortality at trial end**: No significant difference
Secondary Outcome/s	• **Composite of poor neurological function or death at 180 days**: No significant difference
Viva Summary	In a study involving unconscious patients after an OHCA presumed to be of cardiac origin, targeted temperature management at 33°C was compared to 36°C. The primary outcome, all-cause mortality at the end of the trial, was not significantly different, nor was the secondary outcome of a composite of poor neurological function or death at 180 days between the two temperature management approaches.
Study Conclusion	'In unconscious survivors of out-of-hospital cardiac arrest of presumed cardiac cause, hypothermia at a targeted temperature of 33°C did not confer a benefit as compared with a targeted temperature of 36°C.'

TTM (2013): Nielsen N, Wetterslev J, Cronberg T, et al. Targeted temperature management at 33 °C versus 36 °C after cardiac arrest. N Engl J Med. 2013;369(23):2197–2206.

Study Name	TTM 48 (2017)
Population	Unconscious adults after OHCA (presumed cardiac cause)
Intervention	TTM of 33°C for 48 hours vs 24 hours (control)
Primary Outcome/s	• **Favourable neurological outcome at 6 months (CPC 1–2)**: No significant difference
Secondary Outcome/s	• **6-Month mortality, Time to death, Hospital LOS**: No significant difference • **Adverse events, Ventilation time, ICU LOS**: Significantly higher in the 48-hour group
Viva Summary	In a study involving unconscious adults following an OHCA presumed to be of cardiac origin, a comparison was made between two interventions: TTM at 33°C for 48 hours vs TTM for 24 hours. There was no significant difference in favourable neurological outcomes at 6 months between the two groups. Additionally, secondary outcomes such as 6-month mortality, time to death, and hospital LOS did not differ significantly. However, the 48-hour group experienced significantly higher rates of adverse events, longer ventilation times, and longer ICU LOS.
Study Conclusion	'In unconscious survivors from out-of-hospital cardiac arrest admitted to the ICU, targeted temperature management at 33°C for 48 hours did not significantly improve 6-month neurologic outcome compared with targeted temperature management at 33°C for 24 hours. However, the study may have had limited power to detect clinically important differences, and further research may be warranted.'

TTM 48 (2017): Kirkegaard H, Søreide E, de Haas I, et al. Targeted temperature management for 48 vs 24 hours and neurologic outcome after out-of-hospital cardiac arrest: a randomized clinical trial. JAMA. 2017;318(4):341–350.

Study Name	TTM2 (2021)
Population	Unconscious patients post-OHCA
Intervention	Targeted hypothermia (33°C) vs targeted normothermia (<37.5°C)
Primary Outcome/s	• **6-Month all-cause mortality**: No significant difference
Secondary Outcome/s	• **Poor functional outcome at 6 months (mRS 4–6), Quality of life at 6 months**: No significant difference • **Haemodynamically significant arrhythmias**: Significantly higher in 33°C group • **Other complications (e.g., pneumonia, sepsis, bleeding, skin complications)**: No significant difference
Viva Summary	In a study involving unconscious post-OHCA patients, the intervention of targeted hypothermia (33°C) was compared to targeted normothermia (<37.5°C). The primary outcome, which was 6-month all-cause mortality, showed no significant difference between the two groups. Similarly, secondary outcomes such as poor functional outcome and quality of life at 6 months did not differ significantly. However, the 33°C group had a significantly higher incidence of haemodynamically significant arrhythmias, while there was no significant difference in other complications like pneumonia, sepsis, bleeding, and skin complications.
Study Conclusion	'In patients with coma after out-of-hospital cardiac arrest, targeted hypothermia did not lead to a lower incidence of death by 6 months than targeted normothermia.'

TTM2 (2021): Dankiewicz J, Cronberg T, Lilja G, et al. Hypothermia versus normothermia after out-of-hospital cardiac arrest. N Engl J Med. 2021;384(24): 2283–2294.

DELIRIUM

Study Name	Hope-ICU (2013)
Population	Critically ill adults requiring mechanical ventilation
Intervention	Haloperidol 2.5 mg 8-hourly vs placebo (administered for a maximum of 14 days, or until ICU discharge, or until the patient was free from delirium and coma for 2 consecutive days).
Primary Outcome/s	• **Delirium-free and coma-free days in first 14 days**: No significant difference
Secondary Outcome/s	• **28-Day mortality, Hospital LOS, Long QT, Extra-pyramidal symptoms**: No significant difference
Viva Summary	In a study involving critically ill adults needing mechanical ventilation, the use of haloperidol 2.5 mg every 8 hours was compared to a placebo. The primary outcome, which was the number of delirium-free and coma-free days in the first 14 days, was not significantly different between the two groups. Similarly, there were no significant differences in secondary outcomes such as 28-day mortality, hospital LOS, long QT, or extra-pyramidal symptoms.
Study Conclusion	'These results do not support the hypothesis that haloperidol modifies duration of delirium in critically ill patients. Although haloperidol can be used safely in this population of patients, pending the results of trials in progress, the use of intravenous haloperidol should be reserved for short-term management of acute agitation.'

Hope-ICU (2013): Page VJ, Ely EW, Gates S, et al. Effect of intravenous halo-peridol on the duration of delirium and coma in critically ill patients (Hope-ICU): a randomised, double-blind, placebo-controlled trial. Lancet Respir Med. 2013;1(7):515–523.

Study Name	DahLIA (2016)
Population	Adults who continued to require mechanical ventilation due to agitation
Intervention	Addition of dexmedetomidine vs placebo (saline) for up to 7 days
Primary Outcome/s	• **Median ventilator-free hours at 7 days**: Significantly higher in dexmedetomidine group
Secondary Outcome/s	• **Time to extubation, Time to resolution of delirium, Antipsychotic use, Opioid use, Propofol dose**: Significantly lower in dexmedetomidine group
Viva Summary	In a study in adults who remained on mechanical ventilation due to agitation, the addition of dexmedetomidine compared to a placebo (saline) for up to 7 days resulted in significantly more median ventilator-free hours at 7 days. Additionally, secondary outcomes such as time to extubation, time to resolution of delirium, antipsychotic use, opioid use, and propofol dose were significantly reduced in the dexmedetomidine group.
Study Conclusion	'Among patients with agitated delirium receiving mechanical ventilation in the intensive care unit, the addition of dexmedetomidine to standard care compared with standard care alone (placebo) resulted in more ventilator-free hours at 7 days. The findings support the use of dexmedetomidine in patients such as these.'

DahLIA (2016): Reade MC, Eastwood GM, Bellomo R, et al. Effect of dexmedetomidine added to standard care on ventilator-free time in patients with agitated delirium. JAMA. 2016;315(14);1460–1468.

Study Name	AID-ICU (2022)
Population	ICU patients with delirium admitted due to an acute condition
Intervention	Haloperidol 2.5 mg 3 times daily plus 2.5 mg as needed vs placebo until delirium resolved
Primary Outcome/s	• **Number of days alive and out of the hospital at 90 days**: No significant difference
Secondary Outcome/s	• **Mortality at 90 days**: Significantly lower in the haloperidol group (number of patients with missing data was greater than the fragility index) • **Hospital LOS, Days alive without delirium/coma, Serious adverse reactions, Use of rescue medication, Use of open-label antipsychotics**: No significant difference
Viva Summary	In a study involving ICU patients with delirium due to an acute condition, the use of haloperidol 2.5 mg three times daily plus an additional 2.5 mg as needed did not show a significant difference in the number of days alive and out of the hospital at 90 days compared to a placebo. However, the haloperidol group had significantly lower mortality at 90 days, although the number of patients with missing data exceeded the fragility index. Other secondary outcomes such as hospital LOS, days alive without delirium/coma, serious adverse reactions, use of rescue medication, and use of open-label antipsychotics were not significantly different between the two groups.
Study Conclusion	'Among patients in the ICU with delirium, treatment with haloperidol did not lead to a significantly greater number of days alive and out of the hospital at 90 days than placebo.'

AID-ICU (2022): Andersen-Ranberg NC, Poulsen LM, Perner A, Wetterslev J, Estrup S et al. Haloperidol for the treatment of delirium in ICU patients. N Engl J Med. 2022 Dec 29;387(26):2425–2435.

Study Name	Pro-MEDIC (2022)
Population	Adults with an expected ICU stay of >72 hours
Intervention	Enteral melatonin (4 mg at 21:00h) vs placebo for 14 consecutive nights or until ICU discharge
Primary Outcome/s	• **Proportion of delirium-free assessments per patient within 14 days or before ICU discharge**: No significant difference
Secondary Outcome/s	There were no significant differences in various secondary outcomes, including delirium and coma-free days, 90-day mortality, presence of delirium, sleep duration and quality, ICU/hospital LOS, or the need for antipsychotic medications
Viva Summary	In a study involving adult ICU patients with expected stays over 72 hours, the administration of 4 mg of enteral melatonin at 21:00h for 14 consecutive nights or until ICU discharge did not result in a significant difference in delirium-free assessments within 14 days or before ICU discharge. Additionally, various secondary outcomes, including delirium and coma-free days, 90-day mortality, presence of delirium, sleep duration and quality, ICU/hospital LOS, and the need for antipsychotic medications were not significantly different.
Study Conclusion	'Enteral melatonin initiated within 48 h of ICU admission did not reduce the prevalence of delirium compared to placebo. These findings do not support the routine early use of melatonin in the critically ill.'

Pro-MEDIC (2022): Wibrow B, Martinez FE, Myers E, Chapman A, Litton E, Ho KM, Regli et al. Prophylactic melatonin for delirium in intensive care (Pro-MEDIC): a randomized controlled trial. Intensive Care Med. 2022 Apr;48(4):414–425.

SUBARACHNOID HAEMORRHAGE

Study Name	ISAT (2005)
Population	Aneurysmal subarachnoid haemorrhage (SAH)
Intervention	Endovascular coiling vs neurosurgical clipping
Primary Outcome/s	• **Death or dependence (mRS 3–6) at 12 months**: Significantly lower in endovascular coiling group (indicating that coiling led to more patients achieving a better outcome)
Secondary Outcome/s	• **Late rebleeding**: Significantly higher in endovascular coiling group • **Risk of seizures**: Significantly lower in endovascular coiling group
Viva Summary	In a study comparing endovascular coiling and neurosurgical clipping for the treatment of aneurysmal SAH, the primary outcome of death or dependence at 12 months was significantly lower in the endovascular coiling group, indicating better outcomes with coiling. However, it was noted that patients treated with coiling had a significantly higher risk of late rebleeding but a lower risk of seizures compared to those who underwent neurosurgical clipping.
Study Conclusion	'In patients with ruptured intracranial aneurysms suitable for both treatments, endovascular coiling is more likely to result in independent survival at 1 year than neurosurgical clipping; the survival benefit continues for at least 7 years. The risk of late rebleeding is low, but is more common after endovascular coiling than after neurosurgical clipping.'

ISAT (2005): Molyneux AJ, Kerr RSC, Clarke M, et al. International Subarachnoid Aneurysm Trial (ISAT) or neurosurgical clipping versus endovascular coiling in 2143 patients with ruptured intracranial aneurysms: a randomised comparison of effects on survival, dependency, seizures, rebleeding, subgroups, and aneurysm occlusion. Lancet. 2005;366(9488):809–817.

Study Name	MASH-2 (2012)
Population	Adults with aneurysmal SAH
Intervention	IV magnesium sulphate 64 mmol/day vs placebo
Primary Outcome/s	• **Poor outcome (mRS 4–5) or death at 3 months**: No significant difference
Secondary Outcome/s	• **No symptoms at 3 months, Distribution of mRS scores**: No significant difference
Viva Summary	In a study involving adults with aneurysmal SAH, the administration of IV magnesium sulphate at 64 mmol/day did not result in a significant difference in poor outcomes (mRS 4–5) or death at 3 months when compared to a placebo. Additionally, there were no significant differences in secondary outcomes, including the absence of symptoms at 3 months and the distribution of mRS scores.
Study Conclusion	'Intravenous magnesium sulphate does not improve clinical outcome after aneurysmal subarachnoid haemorrhage, therefore routine administration of magnesium cannot be recommended.'

MASH-2 (2012): Mees SMD, Algra A, Vandertop WP, et al. Magnesium for Aneurysmal Subarachnoid Haemorrhage (MASH-2): a randomised placebo-controlled trial. Lancet. 2012;380(9836):44–49.

Study Name	STASH (2014)
Population	Aneurysmal SAH in patients aged 18–65 years
Intervention	Simvastatin 40 mg once a day vs placebo for first 21 days
Primary Outcome/s	• **Distribution of mRS scores at 6 months**: No significant difference
Secondary Outcome/s	• **Hospital LOS, Mortality at discharge, Clinical deterioration related to suspected delayed ischaemia, Serious adverse effects**: No significant difference
Viva Summary	In a study of patients aged 18–65 with aneurysmal SAH, simvastatin 40 mg daily for 21 days did not result in a significant difference in mRS scores at 6 months compared to placebo. Additionally, there were no significant differences in secondary outcomes including hospital LOS, mortality at discharge, clinical deterioration related to suspected delayed ischaemia, or serious adverse effects.
Study Conclusion	'STASH trial did not detect any benefit in the use of simvastatin for long-term or short-term outcome in patients with aneurysmal subarachnoid haemorrhage. Despite demonstrating no safety concerns, we conclude that patients with subarachnoid haemorrhage should not be treated routinely with simvastatin during the acute stages.'

STASH (2014): Kirkpatrick PJ, Turner CL, Smith C, et al. Simvastatin in Aneurysmal Subarachnoid Haemorrhage (STASH): a multicentre randomised phase 3 trial. Lancet Neurol. 2014;13(7):666–675.

Study Name	ULTRA (2021)
Population	Aneurysmal SAH
Intervention	TXA 1-g bolus followed by 1-g infusion every 8 hours from time of diagnosis until aneurysm treatment or 24 hours vs usual care
Primary Outcome/s	• **Good (mRS 0–3) outcome at 6 months**: No significant difference
Secondary Outcome/s	• **Excellent outcome (mRS 0–2) at 6 months**: Significantly lower in TXA group • **6-Month mortality, Serious adverse events, Early rebleeding, DCI, Thromboembolic events**: No significant difference
Viva Summary	In a study involving patients with aneurysmal SAH, the use of TXA did not result in a significant difference in achieving a good outcome (mRS 0–3) at 6 months compared to usual care. However, the likelihood of attaining an excellent outcome (mRS 0–2) at 6 months was significantly lower in the TXA group. There were no significant differences in 6-month mortality, serious adverse events, early rebleeding, DCI, or thromboembolic events between the two groups.
Study Conclusion	'In patients with CT-proven subarachnoid haemorrhage, presumably caused by a ruptured aneurysm, ultra-early, short-term tranexamic acid treatment did not improve clinical outcome at 6 months, as measured by the modified Rankin Scale.'

ULTRA (2021): Post R, Germans MR, Tjerkstra MA, et al. Ultra-early tranexamic acid after subarachnoid haemorrhage (ULTRA): a randomised controlled trial. Lancet. 2020;397(10269):112–118.

TRAUMATIC BRAIN INJURY

Study Name	CRASH (2004)
Population	Head injury with GCS ≤14
Intervention	Early IV methylprednisolone infusion for 48 hours vs placebo
Primary Outcome/s	• **2-Week mortality**: Significantly higher in methylprednisolone group • Trial stopped early
Secondary Outcome/s	• **6-Week mortality ± Severe disability**: Significantly higher in methylprednisolone group
Viva Summary	In a study involving individuals with head injuries and GCS ≤14, the early administration of IV methylprednisolone for 48 hours showed significantly higher 2-week and 6-week mortality rates along with increased severe disability compared to a placebo, leading to the trial being stopped prematurely.
Study Conclusion	'Our results show there is no reduction in mortality with methylprednisolone in the 2 weeks after head injury. The cause of the rise in risk of death within 2 weeks is unclear.'

CRASH (2004): CRASH Trial Collaborators. Effect of intravenous cortico-steroids on death within 14 days in 10008 adults with clinically significant head injury (MRC CRASH trial): randomised placebo-controlled trial. Lancet. 2004;364(9442):1321–1328.

Study Name	DECRA (2011)
Population	TBI with refractory intracranial hypertension
Intervention	Decompressive craniectomy vs standard medical care
Primary Outcome/s	• **Extended Glasgow Outcome Scale (GOS-E) at 6 months**: Significantly worse in the craniectomy group
Secondary Outcome/s	• **Proportion of unfavourable outcomes (GOS-E 1–4) at 6 months**: Significantly higher in the craniectomy group • **Hours of intracranial hypertension, Interventions for increased ICP, Days of mechanical ventilation, ICU LOS**: Significantly lower in craniectomy group • **Mortality at 6 months**: No significant difference
Viva Summary	In a study involving a population with TBI and refractory intracranial hypertension, the outcomes of two interventions were compared: decompressive craniectomy and standard medical care. The primary outcome assessed was the GOS-E at 6 months, which was notably worse in the craniectomy group. Additionally, the craniectomy group exhibited a significantly higher proportion of unfavourable outcomes (GOS-E 1–4) at 6 months. However, this group also showed significantly lower hours of intracranial hypertension, fewer interventions for increased ICP, fewer days of mechanical ventilation, and a shorter ICU LOS. The mortality rate at 6 months did not significantly differ between the two groups.
Study Conclusion	'In adults with severe diffuse traumatic brain injury and refractory intracranial hypertension, early bifrontotemporoparietal decompressive craniectomy decreased intracranial pressure and the length of stay in the ICU but was associated with more unfavorable outcomes.'

DECRA (2011): Cooper DJ, Rosenfeld JV, Murray L, et al. Decompressive craniectomy in diffuse traumatic brain injury. N Engl J Med. 2011;364(16): 1493–1502.

Study Name	Eurotherm3225 (2015)
Population	TBI with high ICP refractory to tier 1 measures
Intervention	Therapeutic hypothermia 32–35°C for 48 hours or until ICP improvement vs standard care
Primary Outcome/s	• **6-Month GOS-E**: Trend towards poorer outcomes in the hypothermia group (terminated after interim analysis)
Secondary Outcome/s	• **6-Month mortality**: Significantly higher in hypothermia group • **Pneumonia in days 1–7, ICU LOS**: No significant difference
Viva Summary	In a study involving patients with TBI and elevated ICP that did not respond to tier 1 treatments, therapeutic hypothermia (32–35°C for 48 hours or until ICP improved) was compared to standard care. The primary outcome, assessed at 6 months using the GOS-E scale, showed a trend towards worse outcomes in the hypothermia group, leading to the trial's termination during interim analysis. Additionally, the hypothermia group had significantly higher 6-month mortality compared to standard care, while there were no significant differences in pneumonia rates during days 1–7 or ICU LOS.
Study Conclusion	'In patients with an intracranial pressure of more than 20 mm Hg after traumatic brain injury, therapeutic hypothermia plus standard care to reduce intracranial pressure did not result in outcomes better than those with standard care alone.'

Eurotherm3235 (2015): Andrews PJD, Sinclair HL, Rodriguez A, et al. Hypothermia for intracranial hypertension after traumatic brain injury. N Engl J Med. 2015;373(25):2403–2412.

Study Name	RESCUEicp (2016)
Population	TBI with abnormal CT and refractory intracranial hypertension
Intervention	Decompressive craniectomy vs medical therapy including barbiturates
Primary Outcome/s	**GOS-E distribution at 6 months**: • **Dead**: Significantly lower in craniectomy group • **Vegetative state (VS), Lower severe disability (LSD), Upper severe disability (USD)**: Significantly higher in craniectomy group • **Moderate disability and good recovery**: No significant difference
Secondary Outcome/s	• **12-Month GOS-E distribution**: Similar between groups
Viva Summary	In a study comparing treatments for TBI with abnormal CT scans and refractory intracranial hypertension, the effects of decompressive craniectomy were compared to medical therapy. At the 6-month mark, the craniectomy group had significantly fewer deaths but significantly more cases of vegetative state, lower severe disability, and upper severe disability compared to the medical therapy group. However, there was no significant difference in the outcomes of moderate disability and good recovery between the two groups. At the 12-month mark, the distribution of outcomes was similar for both groups.
Study Conclusion	'At 6 months, decompressive craniectomy in patients with traumatic brain injury and refractory intracranial hypertension resulted in lower mortality and higher rates of vegetative state, lower severe disability, and upper severe disability than medical care. The rates of moderate disability and good recovery were similar in the two groups.'

RESCUEicp (2016): Hutchinson PJ, Kolias AG, Timfeev IS, et al. Trial of decompressive craniectomy for traumatic intracranial hypertension. N Engl J Med. 2016;375(12):1119–1130.

Study Name	POLAR (2018)
Population	Severe TBI
Intervention	Early induction of hypothermia (33–35°C) vs normothermia (36.5–37.5°C) up to 7 days
Primary Outcome/s	• **6-Month favourable outcome (GOS-E 5–8)**: No significant difference
Secondary Outcome/s	• **GOS-E at 6 months, 6-Month mortality**: No significant difference • **Pneumonia, Incidence of bradycardia**: Significantly higher in hypothermia group
Viva Summary	In a study comparing early induction of hypothermia (33–35°C) with normothermia (36.5–37.5°C) for up to 7 days in patients with severe TBI, there was no significant difference in 6-month favourable outcomes (GOS-E 5–8) or secondary outcomes, including GOS-E at 6 months or 6-month mortality. However, the hypothermia group had a significantly higher incidence of pneumonia and bradycardia.
Study Conclusion	'Among patients with severe traumatic brain injury, early prophylactic hypothermia compared with normothermia did not improve neurologic outcomes at 6 months. These findings do not support the use of early prophylactic hypothermia for patients with severe traumatic brain injury.'

POLAR (2018): Cooper DJ, Nichol AD, Bailey M, et al. Effect of early sustained prophylactic hypothermia on neurologic outcomes among patients with severe traumatic brain injury. JAMA. 2018;320(21):2211–2220.

Study Name	CRASH-3 (2019)
Population	TBI within 3 hours of injury with GCS ≤12 or intracranial bleed on CT
Intervention	TXA (loading dose 1-g over 10 minutes then infusion of 1-g over 8 hours) vs placebo
Primary Outcome/s	• **28-Day in-hospital head injury–associated mortality**: No significant difference • **Subgroup analysis of primary outcome**: In patients with mild to moderate TBI (GCS 9–15), there was significantly reduced mortality in the TXA group
Secondary Outcome/s	• **Vaso-occlusive events, Seizures**: No significant difference
Viva Summary	In a study comparing the use of TXA (1-g loading dose over 10 minutes followed by a 1-g infusion over 8 hours) to a placebo in patients with TBI within 3 hours of injury with GCS ≤12 or intracranial bleed on CT, the primary outcome of 28-day in-hospital head injury–associated mortality showed no significant difference between the two groups. However, a subgroup analysis revealed that in patients with mild to moderate TBI (GCS 9–15), the TXA group had significantly reduced mortality. Secondary outcomes, including vaso-occlusive events and seizures, were not significantly different between the two groups.
Study Conclusion	'Our results show that tranexamic acid is safe in patients with TBI and that treatment within 3 h of injury reduces head injury-related death. Patients should be treated as soon as possible after injury.'

CRASH-3 (2019): The CRASH-3 trial collaborators. Effects of tranexamic acid on death, disability, vascular occlusive events and other morbidities in patients with acute traumatic brain injury (CRASH-3): a randomised, placebo-controlled trial. Lancet. 2019;394(10210):1713–1723.

INTRACEREBRAL HAEMORRHAGE

Study Name	STICH (1998)
Population	Non-traumatic ICH >9 ml with significant neurological impairment
Intervention	Open craniotomy within 12 hours vs medical therapy
Primary Outcome/s	• **6-Month favourable GOS-E**: No significant difference
Secondary Outcome/s	• **6-Month mortality**: No significant difference
Viva Summary	In a study involving patients with non-traumatic ICH >9 ml with significant neurological impairment, the intervention of open craniotomy within 12 hours was compared to medical therapy. The primary outcome, 6-month favourable GOS-E, was not significantly different between the two interventions, and there was no significant difference in 6-month mortality rate.
Study Conclusion	'A trial of early surgery for ICH is feasible. This study represents the largest prospective, randomized series of surgery for ICH. A modest early mortality benefit for surgery is possible, but long-term benefit for surgery was not established in this single-center pilot investigation.'

STICH (1998): Morgenstern LB, Frankowski RF, Shedden P, et al. Surgical Treatment for Intracerebral Haemorrhage (STICH): a single-center, randomized clinical trial. Neurology. 1998;51(5):1359–1363.

Study Name	STICH II (2013)
Population	Spontaneous ICH ≤1 cm from cortex surface
Intervention	Early haematoma evacuation within 12 hours vs initial standard medical therapy
Primary Outcome/s	• **6-Month favourable GOS-E**: No significant difference
Secondary Outcome/s	• **6-Month mortality**: No significant difference
Viva Summary	In a study involving individuals with spontaneous ICH ≤1 cm from the cortex surface, early haematoma evacuation within 12 hours was compared to standard medical therapy. The primary outcome of 6-month favourable GOS-E was not significantly different between the two groups. Additionally, there was no significant difference in 6-month mortality.
Study Conclusion	'The STICH II results confirm that early surgery does not increase the rate of death or disability at 6 months and might have a small but clinically relevant survival advantage for patients with spontaneous superficial intracerebral haemorrhage without intraventricular haemorrhage.'

STICH II (2013): Mendelow AD, Gregson BA, Rowan EN, et al. Early surgery versus initial conservative treatment in patients with spontaneous Supra-Tentorial Intracerebral Haematomas (STICH II): a randomised trial. Lancet. 2013;382(9890):397–408.

Study Name	INTERACT2 (2013)
Population	Spontaneous ICH within 6 hours with elevated systolic blood pressure
Intervention	Intensive BP-lowering (target <140 mmHg within 1 hour) vs standard treatment (target <180 mmHg)
Primary Outcome/s	• **Composite of death or major disability (mRS 3–6) at 90 days**: No significant difference
Secondary Outcome/s	• **mRS, Mortality**: No significant difference • **Reported health-related quality-of-life problems**: Significantly fewer (except mobility)
Viva Summary	In a study comparing intensive blood pressure lowering (target <140 mmHg within 1 hour) to standard treatment (target <180 mmHg) for individuals with spontaneous ICH within 6 hours and elevated systolic blood pressure, there was no significant difference in the primary outcome of death or major disability (mRS 3–6) at 90 days. Similarly, secondary outcomes, including mortality and mRS, were not significantly different between the two groups. However, the intensive BP-lowering group reported significantly fewer health-related quality-of-life problems, except in the domain of mobility.
Study Conclusion	'In patients with intracerebral hemorrhage, intensive lowering of blood pressure did not result in a significant reduction in the rate of the primary outcome of death or severe disability. An ordinal analysis of modified Rankin scores indicated improved functional outcomes with intensive lowering of blood pressure.'

INTERACT2 (2013): Anderson CS, Heeley E, Huang Y, et al. Rapid blood-pressure lowering in patients with acute intracerebral hemorrhage. N Engl J Med. 2013;368(25):2355–2365.

Study Name	STITCH [Trauma] (2015)
Population	Individuals with traumatic ICH, having up to 2 intraparenchymal haemorrhages each of 10 ml or more in volume, and without any extradural or subdural hematoma necessitating surgical intervention
Intervention	Early haematoma evacuation (<12 hours) vs initial conservative management
Primary Outcome/s	• **6-Month unfavourable GOS**: No significant difference (a non-significant benefit of early surgery on the dichotomised GOS favourable vs unfavourable outcome) • Study was halted early due to recruitment difficulties
Secondary Outcome/s	• **6-Month mortality**: Significantly lower in evacuation group
Viva Summary	In a study of patients with traumatic ICH of up to 2 haemorrhages of ≥10 ml, comparison was made between early haematoma evacuation (within 12 hours) and initial conservative management. The primary outcome, which was a 6-month unfavourable GOS, showed no significant difference. However, the secondary outcome, 6-month mortality, was significantly lower in the evacuation group. The study was halted early due to recruitment difficulties.
Study Conclusion	'A larger trial is needed to confirm this potentially very beneficial effect of earlier surgery. In the interim, there is a strong case for operating on patients with traumatic ICH who have a GCS of 9–12. Those who are alert or just confused (GCS 13–15) can probably be watched carefully for any deterioration because there is a safety margin, which diminishes the lower down the GCS the patient descends. Once the GCS has descended below 9, surgical intervention appears to be less effective. A strategy of early surgery is associated with a small, non-significant increase in health care costs, but further analysis using longer-term follow-up data are required to establish better estimates of costs and cost-effectiveness.'

STITCH [Trauma] (2015): Mendelov AD, Gregson BA, Rowan EN, et al. Early surgery versus initial conservative treatment in patients with traumatic intracerebral hemorrhage (STITCH [Trauma]): the first randomized trial. J Neurotrauma. 2015;32(17):1312–1323.

Study Name	ATACH-2 (2016)
Population	Spontaneous ICH <60 cm³ on initial CT scan
Intervention	Intensive BP-lowering (target 110–139 mmHg) vs standard treatment (target 140–179 mmHg) for 24 hours
Primary Outcome/s	• **Death or significant disability (mRS 4–6) at 3 months**: No significant difference
Secondary Outcome/s	• **Haematoma expansion, Neurological deterioration, Mortality**: No significant difference
Viva Summary	In a study comparing intensive blood pressure lowering (target 110–139 mmHg) to standard treatment (target 140–179 mmHg) for 24 hours in individuals with spontaneous ICH <60 cm³ on initial CT, there was no significant difference in the primary outcome of death or significant disability (mRS 4–6) at 3 months. Additionally, secondary outcomes such as haematoma expansion, neurological deterioration, and mortality were not significantly different between the two treatment groups.
Study Conclusion	'The treatment of participants with intracerebral hemorrhage to achieve a target systolic blood pressure of 110 to 139 mm Hg did not result in a lower rate of death or disability than standard reduction to a target of 140 to 179 mm Hg.'

ATACH-2 (2016): Qureshi AI, Palesch YY, Barsan WG, et al. Intensive blood-pressure lowering in patients with acute cerebral haemorrhage. N Engl J Med. 2016;375(11):1033–1043.

Study Name	INCH (2016)
Population	Patients with VKA-related intracranial haemorrhage (VKA-ICH) with INR ≥2
Intervention	Fresh frozen plasma (FFP) vs prothrombin complex concentrate (PCC)
Primary Outcome/s	• **Proportion of patients with INR ≤1.2 within 3 hours of treatment**: Significantly higher in PCC group
Secondary Outcome/s	• The trial was stopped after enrolling 50 patients because emerging evidence indicated a more significant incidence of early haematoma expansion leading to death in the FFP group. There was no comparison of long-term clinical outcomes
Viva Summary	In a study involving patients with VKA-ICH and INR ≥2, the intervention compared FFP to PCC. The primary outcome of proportion of patients achieving an INR ≤1.2 within 3 hours of treatment was significantly greater in the PCC group. The trial was stopped after enrolling 50 patients due to emerging evidence of greater early haematoma expansion and mortality in the FFP group, with no assessment of long-term clinical outcomes.
Study Conclusion	'In patients with VKA-related intracranial hemorrhage, four-factor PCC might be superior to FFP with respect to normalising the INR, and faster INR normalisation seemed to be associated with smaller haematoma expansion. Although an effect of PCC on clinical outcomes remains to be shown, our data favour the use of PCC over FFP in intracranial haemorrhage related to VKA.'

INCH (2016): Steiner T, Poli S, Griebe M, et al. Fresh frozen plasma versus prothrombin complex concentrate in patients with intracranial haemorrhage related to vitamin K antagonists (INCH): a randomised trial. Lancet Neurol. 2016 May;15(6):566–73.

Study Name	TICH-2 (2018)
Population	Spontaneous ICH
Intervention	IV TXA (1-g bolus followed by 1-g over 8 hours) vs placebo
Primary Outcome/s	• **90-Day functional status (mRS)**: No significant difference • Benefit observed for TXA on subgroup analysis if SBP <170 mmHg or baseline haematoma volume 30–60 ml
Secondary Outcome/s	• **90-Day mortality, Hospital LOS**: No significant difference
Viva Summary	In a study comparing TXA (IV 1-g bolus followed by 1-g over 8 hours) to a placebo intervention in patients with spontaneous ICH, the primary outcome of 90-day functional status (measured by mRS) and secondary outcomes, including 90-day mortality and hospital LOS, were not significantly different between the two groups. However, subgroup analysis indicated a potential benefit from TXA in patients with SBP <170 mmHg or a baseline haematoma volume of 30–60 ml.
Study Conclusion	'Functional status 90 days after intracerebral haemorrhage did not differ significantly between patients who received tranexamic acid and those who received placebo, despite a reduction in early deaths and serious adverse events. Larger randomised trials are needed to confirm or refute a clinically significant treatment effect.'

TICH-2 (2018): Sprigg N, Flaherty K, Appleton JP, et al. Tranexamic acid for hyperacute primary IntraCerebral Haemorrhage (TICH-2): an international randomised, placebo-controlled, phase 3 superiority trial. Lancet. 2018;391(10135):2107–2115.

ISCHAEMIC STROKE

Study Name	NINDS (1995)
Population	Acute ischaemic stroke
Intervention	Thrombolysis with t-PA <3 hours onset vs placebo
Primary Outcome/s	• **NIHSS at 24 hours**: No significant difference
Secondary Outcome/s	• **Symptomatic intracerebral haemorrhage within 36 hours after the onset of stroke**: Significantly higher in thrombolysis group • **Favourable functional measures at 3 months (Barthel Index, mRS, GOS, and NIHSS)**: Significantly better in thrombolysis group
Viva Summary	In a study on acute ischaemic stroke, the use of thrombolysis with t-PA within 3 hours of onset was compared to a placebo. The primary outcome, which measured the NIHSS at 24 hours, was not significantly different. However, the secondary outcomes revealed that the thrombolysis group had a significantly higher incidence of symptomatic intracerebral haemorrhage within 36 hours after stroke onset, but also significantly better functional measures at 3 months, as indicated by the Barthel Index, mRS, GOS, and NIHSS.
Study Conclusion	'Despite an increased incidence of symptomatic intracerebral haemorrhage, treatment with intravenous t-PA within three hours of the onset of ischemic stroke improved clinical outcome at three months.'

NINDS (1995): The National Institute of Neurological Disorders and Stroke rt-PA Stroke Study Group. Tissue plasminogen activator for acute ischemic stroke. N Engl J Med. 1995;333(24):1581–1587.

Study Name	DESTINY (2007)
Population	MCA infarction, age 18–60 years
Intervention	Decompressive craniectomy vs conservative treatment
Primary Outcome/s	• **Functional outcome (mRS 0–3) at 6 months**: No significant difference (but non-significant increase) • Trial terminated early (slow recruitment)
Secondary Outcome/s	• **30-Day mortality**: Significantly lower in craniectomy group
Viva Summary	In a study involving individuals aged 18–60 with MCA infarction, decompressive craniectomy was compared to conservative treatment. The primary outcome, which was functional outcome at 6 months (measured by mRS 0–3), was not significantly different between the two groups. However, the craniectomy group had significantly lower 30-day mortality rates compared to the conservative treatment group.
Study Conclusion	'Hemicraniectomy reduces mortality in large hemispheric stroke. With 32 patients included, the primary end point failed to demonstrate statistical superiority of hemicraniectomy, and the projected sample size was calculated to 188 patients. Despite this failure to meet the primary end point, the steering committee decided to terminate the trial in light of the results of the joint analysis of the 3 European hemicraniectomy trials.'

DESTINY (2007): Jüttler E, Schwab S, Schmiedek P, et al. Decompressive surgery for the treatment of malignant infarction of the middle cerebral artery (DESTINY): a randomized, controlled trial. Stroke. 2007;38(9):2518–2525.

Study Name	DECIMAL (2007)
Population	Malignant MCA infarction, ages 18–55 years
Intervention	Decompressive hemicraniectomy vs conservative management
Primary Outcome/s	• **Favourable functional outcome (mRS ≤3) at 6 and 12 months**: No significant difference • When using a higher disability threshold (mRS ≤4), patients who had a decompressive hemicraniectomy had significantly better outcomes at 6 and 12 months, based on non-dichotomised mRS scores
Secondary Outcome/s	• **6-Month and 12-Month mortality**: Significantly lower in craniectomy group • **Subgroup analysis**: Younger age correlated with a more favourable mRS at 6 months in the hemicraniectomy group
Viva Summary	In a study involving individuals aged 18–55 with malignant MCA infarction, a comparison was made between decompressive hemicraniectomy and conservative management. The primary outcome, which assessed favourable functional outcomes (mRS ≤3) at 6 and 12 months, was not significantly different between the two groups. However, when a higher disability threshold (mRS ≤4) was considered, patients who underwent decompressive hemicraniectomy had significantly better outcomes at both 6 and 12 months based on non-dichotomised mRS scores. Additionally, the craniectomy group had lower mortality rates at both time points, and subgroup analysis revealed that younger patients in the hemicraniectomy group had more favourable outcomes at 6 months.
Study Conclusion	'In this trial, early decompressive craniectomy increased by more than half the number of patients with moderate disability and very significantly reduced (by more than half) the mortality rate compared with that after medical therapy.'

DECIMAL (2007): Vahedi K, Vicaut E, Mateo J, et al. Sequential-design, multicenter, randomized, controlled trial of early decompressive craniectomy in malignant middle cerebral artery infarction (DECIMAL Trial). Stroke. 2007;38(9):2506–2517.

Study Name	HAMLET (2009)
Population	Space-occupying hemispheric infarction
Intervention	Decompressive craniectomy vs conservative treatment within 4 days
Primary Outcome/s	• **mRS at 1 year (good [0–3] or poor [4–6] outcome)**: No significant difference
Secondary Outcome/s	• **Mortality**: Significantly lower • A meta-analysis, which included the DESTINY and DECIMAL trials, demonstrated a decrease in unfavourable outcomes and case fatality rates
Viva Summary	In a study comparing decompressive craniectomy to conservative treatment for space-occupying hemispheric infarction within 4 days, there was no significant difference in good or poor outcomes (measured by mRS) at 1 year. However, mortality rates were significantly lower in the decompressive craniectomy group. Additionally, a meta-analysis that included the DESTINY and DECIMAL trials showed a reduction in unfavourable outcomes and case fatality rates.
Study Conclusion	'Surgical decompression reduces case fatality and poor outcome in patients with space-occupying infarctions who are treated within 48 h of stroke onset. There is no evidence that this operation improves functional outcome when it is delayed for up to 96 h after stroke onset. The decision to perform the operation should depend on the emphasis patients and relatives attribute to survival and dependency.'

HAMLET (2009): Hofmeijer J, Kappelle LJ, Algra A, et al. Surgical decompression for space-occupying cerebral infarction (the hemicraniectomy after middle cerebral artery infarction with life-threatening edema trial [HAMLET]): a multicentre, open, randomised trial. Lancet Neurol. 2009;8(4):326–333.

Study Name	DESTINY II (2011)
Population	Malignant MCA infarction, age ≥61 years
Intervention	Decompressive hemicraniectomy <48 hours onset vs conservative management
Primary Outcome/s	• **mRS 0–4 at 6 months**: Significantly higher in hemicraniectomy group
Secondary Outcome/s	• **1-Year mortality**: Significantly lower in hemicraniectomy group • No patient who survived had a score of 0–2 on the mRS
Viva Summary	In a study of patients ≥61 years with malignant MCA infarction, those who underwent decompressive hemicraniectomy within 48 hours of onset compared to conservative management had significantly better outcomes at 6 months, with a higher proportion having mRS scores of 0–4. Additionally, the hemicraniectomy group had a significantly lower 1-year mortality rate, though none of the surviving patients had the most favourable mRS scores of 0–2.
Study Conclusion	'The results of this trial are expected to directly influence decision making in these patients.'

DESTINY II (2011): Jüttler E, Bösel J, Amiri H, et al. DESTINY II: DEcompressive Surgery for the Treatment of malignant INfarction of the middle cerebral arterY II. Int J Stroke. 2011;6(1):79–86.

Study Name	IST-3 (2012)
Population	Acute ischaemic stroke
Intervention	t-PA vs placebo <6 hours of stroke
Primary Outcome/s	• **Oxford Handicap Scale (OHS) 0–2 at 6 months**: No significant difference • Did not meet recruitment numbers
Secondary Outcome/s	• **7-Day mortality**: Significantly higher in t-PA group • **6-Month mortality**: Significantly lower in t-PA group
Viva Summary	In a study comparing t-PA to a placebo for acute ischaemic stroke within 6 hours of onset, the primary outcome of achieving an Oxford Handicap Scale score of 0–2 at 6 months was not significantly different. However, the t-PA group had significantly higher 7-day mortality and significantly lower 6-month mortality compared to the placebo group.
Study Conclusion	'For the types of patients recruited in IST-3, despite the early hazards, thrombolysis within 6 h improved functional outcome. Benefit did not seem to be diminished in elderly patients.'

IST-3 (2012): The IST-3 Collaborative Group. The benefits and harms of intravenous thrombolysis with recombinant tissue plasminogen activator within 6 h of acute ischaemic stroke (the Third International Stroke Trial [IST-3]): a randomised controlled trial. Lancet. 2012;379(9834):2352–2363.

Study Name	EuroHYP-1 (2014)
Population	Acute ischaemic stroke
Intervention	Cooling to target 34–35°C within 6 hours and maintained for 24 hours vs standard care
Primary Outcome/s	• **mRS at 91 days**: No significant difference
Secondary Outcome/s	• Trial was stopped early due to recruitment difficulty/ funding
Viva Summary	In a study comparing cooling to 34–35°C within 6 hours of an acute ischaemic stroke and maintaining this for 24 hours versus standard care, there was no significant difference in the primary outcome of mRS at 91 days. The trial was stopped prematurely due to challenges in recruitment and funding issues.
Study Conclusion	'With 750 patients per intervention group, this trial has 90% power to detect 7% absolute improvement at the 5% significance level.'

EuroHYP-1 (2014): van der Worp HB, Macleod MR, Bath PMW, et al. Euro-HYP-1: European multicenter, randomized, phase III clinical trial of therapeutic hypothermia plus best medical treatment vs. best medical treatment alone for acute ischemic stroke. Int J Stroke. 2014;9(5):642–645.

Study Name	DAWN (2018)
Population	Acute ischaemic stroke, 6–24 hours from onset
Intervention	Thrombectomy vs standard care alone
Primary Outcome/s	• **Utility-weighted mRS at 90 days**: Significantly better in thrombectomy group • **Functional independence at 90 days (mRS 0–2)**: Significantly higher in thrombectomy group
Secondary Outcome/s	• **NIHSS decrease, Vessel recanalisation**: Significantly higher in thrombectomy group • **Infarct volume/change**: Significantly lower in thrombectomy group • **90-Day mortality**: No significant difference
Viva Summary	In a study involving individuals with acute ischaemic stroke who were 6–24 hours from onset, thrombectomy was compared to standard care. The thrombectomy group had significantly better utility-weighted mRS and functional independence at 90 days (mRS 0–2). Secondary outcomes also favoured the thrombectomy group, with a higher NIHSS decrease, vessel recanalisation, and lower infarct volume/change, although 90-day mortality was not significantly different.
Study Conclusion	'Among patients with acute stroke who had last been known to be well 6 to 24 hours earlier and who had a mismatch between clinical deficit and infarct, outcomes for disability at 90 days were better with thrombectomy plus standard care than with standard care alone.'

DAWN (2018): Nogueira RG, Jadhav AP, Haussen DC, et al. Thrombectomy 6 to 24 hours after stroke with a mismatch between deficit and infarct. N Engl J Med. 2018;378(1):11–21.

Study Name	DEFUSE 3 (2018)
Population	Proximal ICA/MCA stroke 6–16 hours from onset with initial infarct <70 ml and ratio of ischaemic tissue:infarct volume ≥1.8
Intervention	Thrombectomy vs standard medical therapy
Primary Outcome/s	• **Functional outcome (mRS) at 90 days**: Significantly more favourable in thrombectomy group
Secondary Outcome/s	• **Functional independence (mRS 0–2) at 90 days**: Significantly higher in thrombectomy group • **Mortality at 90 days, Symptomatic intracranial haemorrhage, Adverse events**: No significant difference
Viva Summary	In a study involving patients with proximal ICA/MCA stroke occurring 6–16 hours from onset, where the initial infarct volume was less than 70 ml and the ischaemic tissue:infarct volume ratio was ≥1.8, thrombectomy was compared to standard medical therapy. The primary outcome, functional outcome (measured by mRS) at 90 days, was significantly better in the thrombectomy group. Additionally, the thrombectomy group had significantly higher rates of functional independence (mRS 0–2) at 90 days. There was no significant difference in mortality at 90 days, symptomatic intracranial haemorrhage, or adverse events between the two groups.
Study Conclusion	'Endovascular thrombectomy for ischemic stroke 6 to 16 hours after a patient was last known to be well plus standard medical therapy resulted in better functional outcomes than standard medical therapy alone among patients with proximal middle-cerebral-artery or internal-carotid-artery occlusion and a region of tissue that was ischemic but not yet infarcted.'

DEFUSE 3 (2018): Albers GW, Marks MP, Kemp S, et al. Thrombectomy for stroke at 6 to 16 hours with selection by perfusion imaging. N Engl J Med. 2018;378(8):708–718.

STATUS EPILEPTICUS

Study Name	HYBERNATUS (2016)
Population	Convulsive status epilepticus receiving mechanical ventilation
Intervention	Hypothermia (target temperature 32–34°C) for 24 hours vs standard care only
Primary Outcome/s	• **Good functional outcome (GOS score of 5) at 90 days**: No significant difference
Secondary Outcome/s	• **Mortality, Seizure duration, LOS, Refractory status epilepticus**: No significant difference • **Progression of EEG-confirmed status epilepticus on day 1**: Significantly lower in hypothermia group
Viva Summary	In a study involving convulsive status epilepticus patients on mechanical ventilation, the use of hypothermia at a target temperature of 32–34°C for 24 hours did not result in a significant difference in achieving a good functional outcome at 90 days compared to standard care. Additionally, there were no significant differences in mortality, seizure duration, LOS, or refractory status epilepticus between the two groups. However, the hypothermia group did exhibit a significantly lower progression of EEG-confirmed status epilepticus on the first day of treatment.
Study Conclusion	'In this trial, induced hypothermia added to standard care was not associated with significantly better 90-day outcomes than standard care alone in patients with convulsive status epilepticus.'

HYBERNATUS (2016): Legriel S, Lemiale V, Schenck M, et al. Hypothermia for neuroprotection in convulsive status epilepticus. N Engl J Med. 2016;375(25):2457–2467.

MENINGITIS

Study Name	Brouwer et al. (2015)
Population	Acute bacterial meningitis (children and adults)
Intervention	Cochrane review of corticosteroids
Key Findings	• Corticosteroids did not significantly reduce overall mortality. Subgroup analysis showed a reduction in mortality in cases of *Streptococcus pneumoniae* meningitis but not in those with *Haemophilus influenzae* or *Neisseria meningitidis* meningitis • Corticosteroids were significantly associated with lower rates of severe hearing loss, any hearing loss, and neurological sequelae • Corticosteroids significantly reduced severe hearing loss in children with *H. influenzae* meningitis but not in those with meningitis caused by non-*Haemophilus* species meningitis • In high-income countries, corticosteroids significantly reduced hearing loss and short-term neurological sequelae. No beneficial effect of corticosteroids was observed in low-income countries
Viva Summary	A Cochrane review indicated that corticosteroids significantly reduce hearing loss, severe hearing loss, and neurological sequelae in acute bacterial meningitis. Mortality rates were significantly lower for *S. pneumoniae* meningitis but unchanged for *N. meningitidis* or *H. influenzae* meningitis. In children with *H. influenzae* meningitis, a notable reduction in severe hearing loss was observed. The benefits of corticosteroids, including reduced hearing loss and neurological sequelae, were more pronounced in high-income countries, with no marked benefits noted in low-income countries.
Study Conclusion	'Corticosteroids significantly reduced hearing loss and neurological sequelae, but did not reduce overall mortality. Data support the use of corticosteroids in patients with bacterial meningitis in high-income countries. We found no beneficial effect in low-income countries.'

Brouwer et al. (2015): Brouwer MC, McIntyre P, Prasad K, et al. Corticosteroids for acute bacterial meningitis. Cochrane Database Syst Rev. 2015;2015(9): CD004405.

SUMMARY

1. **ABC (2008):** In a study involving mechanically ventilated and sedated patients, the intervention group underwent an SAT followed by an SBT, while the control group received an SBT alone. The intervention group had significantly more VFDs by day 28, lower ICU/hospital LOS, and lower 1-year mortality. However, the intervention group also had a higher rate of self-extubation, with no significant difference in reintubation rates, even after self-extubation.

2. **SLEAP (2012):** In a study involving mechanically ventilated patients sedated with opioids and/or benzodiazepines, the primary outcome of days to extubation was not significantly different between the group receiving daily sedation interruption and the group with no planned sedation interruption. However, in a subgroup analysis of trauma and surgical patients, the interruption group experienced significantly fewer days to extubation. Additionally, the interruption group required higher doses of sedatives/analgesics and resulted in a higher nurse/respiratory therapist clinical workload. There were no significant differences in ICU LOS, rates of delirium, or unintentional device removal between the two groups.

3. **MIDEX-PRODEX (2012):** Two trials, MIDEX and PRODEX, compared dexmedetomidine with midazolam and propofol in adult ICU patients on prolonged mechanical ventilation. Dexmedetomidine was found to be non-inferior to both midazolam and propofol in maintaining target sedation levels. However, the duration of mechanical ventilation was significantly shorter with dexmedetomidine compared to midazolam, but not propofol. Dexmedetomidine also led to a significantly shorter median time to extubation and improved patient outcomes in terms of pain communication, arousability, and cooperation, compared to both alternatives. However, it was associated with a higher incidence of hypotension and bradycardia than midazolam. There was no significant difference in ICU LOS between the groups.

4. **TTM (2013):** In a study involving unconscious patients after an OHCA presumed to be of cardiac origin, targeted temperature management at 33°C was compared to 36°C. The primary outcome, all-cause mortality at the end of the trial, was not significantly

different, nor was the secondary outcome of a composite of poor neurological function or death at 180 days between the two temperature management approaches.

5. **TTM 48 (2017):** In a study involving unconscious adults following an OHCA presumed to be of cardiac origin, a comparison was made between two interventions: TTM at 33°C for 48 hours vs TTM for 24 hours. There was no significant difference in favourable neurological outcomes at 6 months between the two groups. Additionally, secondary outcomes such as 6-month mortality, time to death, and hospital LOS did not differ significantly. However, the 48-hour group experienced significantly higher rates of adverse events, longer ventilation times, and longer ICU LOS.

6. **TTM2 (2021):** In a study involving unconscious post-OHCA patients, the intervention of targeted hypothermia (33°C) was compared to targeted normothermia (<37.5°C). The primary outcome, which was 6-month all-cause mortality, showed no significant difference between the two groups. Similarly, secondary outcomes such as poor functional outcome and quality of life at 6 months did not differ significantly. However, the 33°C group had a significantly higher incidence of haemodynamically significant arrhythmias, while there was no significant difference in other complications like pneumonia, sepsis, bleeding, and skin complications.

7. **HOPE-ICU (2013):** In a study involving critically ill adults needing mechanical ventilation, the use of haloperidol 2.5 mg every 8 hours was compared to a placebo. The primary outcome, which was the number of delirium-free and coma-free days in the first 14 days, was not significantly different between the two groups. Similarly, there were no significant differences in secondary outcomes such as 28-day mortality, hospital LOS, long QT, or extrapyramidal symptoms.

8. **DahLIA (2016):** In a study on adults who remained on mechanical ventilation due to agitation, the addition of dexmedetomidine compared to a placebo (saline) for up to 7 days resulted in significantly more median ventilator-free hours at 7 days. Additionally, secondary outcomes such as time to extubation, time to resolution of delirium, antipsychotic use, opioid use, and propofol dose were significantly reduced in the dexmedetomidine group.

9. **AID-ICU (2022):** In a study involving ICU patients with delirium due to an acute condition, the use of haloperidol 2.5 mg three times daily plus an additional 2.5 mg as needed did not show a significant difference in the number of days alive and out of the hospital at 90 days compared to a placebo. However, the haloperidol group had significantly lower mortality at 90 days, although the number of patients with missing data exceeded the fragility index. Other secondary outcomes such as hospital LOS, days alive without delirium/coma, serious adverse reactions, use of rescue medication, and use of open-label antipsychotics were not significantly different between the two groups.

10. **PRO-MEDIC (2022):** In a study involving adult ICU patients with expected stays over 72 hours, the administration of 4 mg of enteral melatonin at 21:00h for 14 consecutive nights or until ICU discharge did not result in a significant difference in delirium-free assessments within 14 days or before ICU discharge. Additionally, various secondary outcomes, including delirium and coma-free days, 90-day mortality, presence of delirium, sleep duration and quality, ICU/hospital LOS, and the need for antipsychotic medications were not significantly different.

11. **ISAT (2005):** In a study comparing endovascular coiling and neurosurgical clipping for the treatment of aneurysmal SAH, the primary outcome of death or dependence at 12 months was significantly lower in the endovascular coiling group, indicating better outcomes with coiling. However, it was noted that patients treated with coiling had a significantly higher risk of late rebleeding but a lower risk of seizures compared to those who underwent neurosurgical clipping.

12. **MASH-2 (2012):** In a study involving adults with aneurysmal SAH, the administration of IV magnesium sulphate at 64 mmol/day did not result in a significant difference in poor outcomes (mRS 4–5) or death at 3 months when compared to a placebo. Additionally, there were no significant differences in secondary outcomes, including the absence of symptoms at 3 months and the distribution of mRS scores.

13. **STASH (2014):** In a study of patients aged 18–65 with aneurysmal SAH, simvastatin 40 mg daily for 21 days did not result in a significant difference in mRS scores at 6 months compared to placebo. Additionally, there were no significant differences

in secondary outcomes including hospital LOS, mortality at discharge, clinical deterioration related to suspected delayed ischaemia, or serious adverse effects.

14. **ULTRA (2021):** In a study involving patients with aneurysmal SAH, the use of TXA did not result in a significant difference in achieving a good outcome (mRS 0–3) at 6 months compared to usual care. However, the likelihood of attaining an excellent outcome (mRS 0–2) at 6 months was significantly lower in the TXA group. There were no significant differences in 6-month mortality, serious adverse events, early rebleeding, DCI, or thromboembolic events between the two groups.

15. **CRASH (2004):** In a study involving individuals with head injuries and GCS ≤14, the early administration of IV methylprednisolone for 48 hours showed significantly higher 2-week and 6-week mortality rates along with increased severe disability compared to a placebo, leading to the trial being stopped prematurely.

16. **DECRA (2011):** In a study involving a population with TBI and refractory intracranial hypertension, the outcomes of two interventions were compared: decompressive craniectomy and standard medical care. The primary outcome assessed was the GOS-E at 6 months, which was notably worse in the craniectomy group. Additionally, the craniectomy group exhibited a significantly higher proportion of unfavourable outcomes (GOS-E 1–4) at 6 months. However, this group also showed significantly lower hours of intracranial hypertension, fewer interventions for increased ICP, fewer days of mechanical ventilation, and a shorter ICU LOS. The mortality rate at 6 months did not significantly differ between the two groups.

17. **Eurotherm3225 (2015):** In a study involving patients with TBI and elevated ICP that did not respond to tier 1 treatments, therapeutic hypothermia (32–35°C for 48 hours or until ICP improved) was compared to standard care. The primary outcome, assessed at 6 months using the GOS-E scale, showed a trend towards worse outcomes in the hypothermia group, leading to the trial's termination during interim analysis. Additionally, the hypothermia group had significantly higher 6-month mortality compared to standard care, while there were no significant differences in pneumonia rates during days 1–7 or ICU LOS.

18. **RESCUEicp (2016):** In a study comparing treatments for TBI with abnormal CT scans and refractory intracranial hypertension, the effects of decompressive craniectomy were compared to medical therapy. At the 6-month mark, the craniectomy group had significantly fewer deaths but significantly more cases of vegetative state, lower severe disability, and upper severe disability compared to the medical therapy group. However, there was no significant difference in the outcomes of moderate disability and good recovery between the two groups. At the 12-month mark, the distribution of outcomes was similar for both groups.

19. **POLAR (2018):** In a study comparing early induction of hypothermia (33–35°C) with normothermia (36.5–37.5°C) for up to 7 days in patients with severe TBI, there was no significant difference in 6-month favourable outcomes (GOS-E 5–8) or secondary outcomes, including GOS-E at 6 months or 6-month mortality. However, the hypothermia group had a significantly higher incidence of pneumonia and bradycardia.

20. **CRASH-3 (2019):** In a study comparing the use of TXA (1-g loading dose over 10 minutes followed by a 1-g infusion over 8 hours) to a placebo in patients with TBI within 3 hours of injury with GCS ≤12 or intracranial bleed on CT, the primary outcome of 28-day in-hospital head injury–associated mortality showed no significant difference between the two groups. However, a subgroup analysis revealed that in patients with mild to moderate TBI (GCS 9–15), the TXA group had significantly reduced mortality. Secondary outcomes, including vaso-occlusive events and seizures, were not significantly different between the two groups.

21. **STICH (1998):** In a study involving patients with non-traumatic ICH >9 ml with significant neurological impairment, the intervention of open craniotomy within 12 hours was compared to medical therapy. The primary outcome, 6-month favourable GOS-E, was not significantly different between the two interventions, and there was no significant difference in 6-month mortality rate.

22. **STICH II (2013):** In a study involving individuals with spontaneous ICH ≤1 cm from the cortex surface, early haematoma evacuation within 12 hours was compared to standard medical therapy. The primary outcome of 6-month favourable GOS-E was not significantly different between the two groups. Additionally, there was no significant difference in 6-month mortality.

23. **INTERACT2 (2013):** In a study comparing intensive blood pressure lowering (target <140 mmHg within 1 hour) to standard treatment (target <180 mmHg) for individuals with spontaneous ICH within 6 hours and elevated systolic blood pressure, there was no significant difference in the primary outcome of death or major disability (mRS 3–6) at 90 days. Similarly, secondary outcomes, including mortality and mRS, were not significantly different between the two groups. However, the intensive BP-lowering group reported significantly fewer health-related quality-of-life problems, except in the domain of mobility.

24. **STITCH [Trauma] (2015):** In a study of patients with traumatic ICH of up to 2 haemorrhages of ≥10 ml, comparison was made between early haematoma evacuation (within 12 hours) and initial conservative management. The primary outcome, which was a 6-month unfavourable GOS, showed no significant difference. However, the secondary outcome, 6-month mortality, was significantly lower in the evacuation group. The study was halted early due to recruitment difficulties.

25. **ATACH-2 (2016):** In a study comparing intensive blood pressure lowering (target 110–139 mmHg) to standard treatment (target 140–179 mmHg) for 24 hours in individuals with spontaneous ICH <60 cm^3 on initial CT, there was no significant difference in the primary outcome of death or significant disability (mRS 4–6) at 3 months. Additionally, secondary outcomes such as haematoma expansion, neurological deterioration, and mortality were not significantly different between the two treatment groups.

26. **INCH (2016):** In a study involving patients with VKA-ICH and INR ≥2, the intervention compared FFP to PCC. The primary outcome of proportion of patients achieving an INR ≤1.2 within 3 hours of treatment was significantly greater in the PCC group. The trial was stopped after enrolling 50 patients due to emerging evidence of greater early haematoma expansion and mortality in the FFP group, with no assessment of long-term clinical outcomes.

27. **TICH-2 (2018):** In a study comparing TXA (IV 1-g bolus followed by 1 g over 8 hours) to a placebo intervention in patients with spontaneous ICH, the primary outcome of 90-day functional status (measured by mRS) and secondary outcomes, including 90-day mortality and hospital LOS, were not significantly different

between the two groups. However, subgroup analysis indicated potential benefit from TXA in patients with SBP <170 mmHg or a baseline haematoma volume of 30–60 ml.

28. **NINDS (1995):** In a study on acute ischaemic stroke, the use of thrombolysis with t-PA within 3 hours of onset was compared to a placebo. The primary outcome, which measured the NIHSS at 24 hours, was not significantly different. However, the secondary outcomes revealed that the thrombolysis group had a significantly higher incidence of symptomatic intracerebral haemorrhage within 36 hours after stroke onset, but also significantly better functional measures at 3 months, as indicated by the Barthel Index, mRS, GOS, and NIHSS.

29. **DESTINY (2007):** In a study involving individuals aged 18–60 with MCA infarction, decompressive craniectomy was compared to conservative treatment. The primary outcome, which was functional outcome at 6 months (measured by mRS 0–3), was not significantly different between the two groups. However, the craniectomy group had significantly lower 30-day mortality rates compared to the conservative treatment group.

30. **DECIMAL (2007):** In a study involving individuals aged 18–55 with malignant MCA infarction, a comparison was made between decompressive hemicraniectomy and conservative management. The primary outcome, which assessed favourable functional outcomes (mRS ≤3) at 6 and 12 months, was not significantly different between the two groups. However, when a higher disability threshold (mRS ≤4) was considered, patients who underwent decompressive hemicraniectomy had significantly better outcomes at both 6 and 12 months based on non-dichotomised mRS scores. Additionally, the craniectomy group had lower mortality rates at both time points, and subgroup analysis revealed that younger patients in the hemicraniectomy group had more favourable outcomes at 6 months.

31. **HAMLET (2009):** In a study comparing decompressive craniectomy to conservative treatment for space-occupying hemispheric infarction within 4 days, there was no significant difference in good or poor outcomes (measured by mRS) at 1 year. However, mortality rates were significantly lower in the decompressive craniectomy group. Additionally, a meta-analysis that included the DESTINY and DECIMAL trials showed a reduction in unfavourable outcomes and case fatality rates.

32. **DESTINY II (2011):** In a study of patients ≥61 years with malignant MCA infarction, those who underwent decompressive hemicraniectomy within 48 hours of onset compared to conservative management had significantly better outcomes at 6 months, with a higher proportion having mRS scores of 0–4. Additionally, the hemicraniectomy group had a significantly lower 1-year mortality rate, though none of the surviving patients had the most favourable mRS scores of 0–2.

33. **IST-3 (2012):** In a study comparing t-PA to a placebo for acute ischaemic stroke within 6 hours of onset, the primary outcome of achieving an Oxford Handicap Scale score of 0–2 at 6 months was not significantly different. However, the t-PA group had significantly higher 7-day mortality and significantly lower 6-month mortality compared to the placebo group.

34. **EuroHYP-1 (2014):** In a study comparing cooling to 34–35°C within 6 hours of an acute ischaemic stroke and maintaining this for 24 hours versus standard care, there was no significant difference in the primary outcome of mRS at 91 days. The trial was stopped prematurely due to challenges in recruitment and funding issues.

35. **DAWN (2018):** In a study involving individuals with acute ischaemic stroke who were 6–24 hours from onset, thrombectomy was compared to standard care. The thrombectomy group had significantly better utility-weighted mRS and functional independence at 90 days (mRS 0–2). Secondary outcomes also favoured the thrombectomy group, with a higher NIHSS decrease, vessel recanalisation, and lower infarct volume/change, although 90-day mortality was not significantly different.

36. **DEFUSE 3 (2018):** In a study involving patients with proximal ICA/MCA stroke occurring 6–16 hours from onset, where the initial infarct volume was less than 70 ml and the ischaemic tissue:infarct volume ratio was ≥1.8, thrombectomy was compared to standard medical therapy. The primary outcome, functional outcome (measured by mRS) at 90 days, was significantly better in the thrombectomy group. Additionally, the thrombectomy group had significantly higher rates of functional independence (mRS 0–2) at 90 days. There was no significant difference in mortality at 90 days, symptomatic intracranial haemorrhage, or adverse events between the two groups.

37. **HYBERNATUS (2016):** In a study involving convulsive status epilepticus patients on mechanical ventilation, the use of hypothermia at a target temperature of 32–34°C for 24 hours did not result in a significant difference in achieving a good functional outcome at 90 days compared to standard care. Additionally, there were no significant differences in mortality, seizure duration, LOS, or refractory status epilepticus between the two groups. However, the hypothermia group did exhibit a significantly lower progression of EEG-confirmed status epilepticus on the first day of treatment.

38. **Brouwer et al. (2015):** A Cochrane review indicated that corticosteroids significantly reduce hearing loss, severe hearing loss, and neurological sequelae in acute bacterial meningitis. Mortality rates were significantly lower for *S. pneumoniae* meningitis but unchanged for *N. meningitidis* or *H. influenzae* meningitis. In children with *H. influenzae* meningitis, a notable reduction in severe hearing loss was observed. The benefits of corticosteroids, including reduced hearing loss and neurological sequelae, were more pronounced in high-income countries, with no marked benefits noted in low-income countries.

CHAPTER 4
GASTROINTESTINAL, NUTRITION, AND LIVER DISEASE

NUTRITION

Study Name	TICACOS (2011)
Population	Critically ill adult patients on mechanical ventilation with expected ICU stay >3 days
Intervention	Nutritional support guided by daily resting energy expenditure (REE) measurements vs weight-based regimen (25 kcal/kg/day)
Primary Outcome/s	• **Hospital mortality**: No significant difference
Secondary Outcome/s	• **Energy delivered, Receipt of parenteral nutrition in first 3 days, Duration of ventilation, ICU LOS**: Significantly higher in REE group
Viva Summary	In a study involving critically ill adult patients requiring mechanical ventilation for more than 3 days, two nutritional support approaches were compared: one guided by daily REE measurements and the other based on a fixed weight-based regimen of 25 kcal/kg/day. The primary outcome, hospital mortality, was not significantly different between the two groups. However, secondary outcome analysis showed that the REE-guided group received more energy, had a higher rate of parenteral nutrition in the first 3 days, and experienced longer durations of ventilation and ICU LOS compared to the weight-based regimen group.

(Continued)

(Continued)

Study Name	TICACOS (2011)
Study Conclusion	'In this single-center pilot study a bundle comprising actively supervised nutritional intervention and providing near target energy requirements based on repeated energy measurements was achievable in a general ICU and may be associated with lower hospital mortality.'

TICACOS (2011): Singer P, Anbar R, Cohen J, et al. The tight calorie control study (TICACOS): a prospective, randomized, controlled pilot study of nutritional support in critically ill patients. Intensive Care Med. 2011;37(4): 601–609.

Study Name	OMEGA (2011)
Population	Adults with acute lung injury requiring mechanical ventilation
Intervention	Enteral supplementation of n-3 fatty acids + γ-linolenic acids + antioxidants vs isocaloric control
Primary Outcome/s	• **VFDs to day 28**: Significantly lower in the intervention group
Secondary Outcome/s	• **Non-pulmonary organ failure–free days, ICU-free days**: Significantly lower in the intervention group • **Days of diarrhoea**: Significantly higher in the intervention group • **60-Day mortality**: Higher in the intervention group, though the statistical significance was borderline ($p = 0.054$) • The study was stopped early for futility/potential harm
Viva Summary	In a study involving adults with acute lung injury requiring mechanical ventilation, the effects of enteral supplementation of n-3 fatty acids, γ-linolenic acids, and antioxidants were compared with an isocaloric control group. The intervention group had significantly fewer VFDs to day 28, experienced significantly lower non-pulmonary organ failure–free days and ICU-free days, and also had more days with diarrhoea. Additionally, there was a higher 60-day mortality rate in the intervention group, although the statistical significance was borderline. The study was halted prematurely due to concerns about potential harm or futility.
Study Conclusion	'Twice-daily enteral supplementation of n-3 fatty acids, γ-linolenic acid, and antioxidants did not improve the primary end point of ventilator-free days or other clinical outcomes in patients with acute lung injury and may be harmful.'

OMEGA (2011): Rice TW, Wheeler AP, Thompson BT, deBoisblanc BP et al.; NIH NHLBI Acute Respiratory Distress Syndrome Network of Investigators. Enteral omega-3 fatty acid, gamma-linolenic acid, and antioxidant supplementation in acute lung injury. JAMA. 2011 Oct 12;306(14):1574–1581.

Study Name	EPaNIC (2011)
Population	Critically ill adults
Intervention	Late parenteral nutrition (PN) on day 8 vs early PN on day 3
Primary Outcome/s	• **ICU LOS**: Significantly shorter in late PN group • **Discharged alive from ICU within 8 days, Incidence of hypoglycaemia**: Significantly higher in late PN group • **Mortality**: No significant difference
Secondary Outcome/s	• **New infection, Duration of mechanical ventilation, Duration of RRT, Hospital LOS, Health care cost**: Significantly lower in late PN group • **Functional status on hospital discharge**: No significant difference
Viva Summary	In a study comparing the timing of PN in critically ill adults, it was found that administering PN on day 8, rather than on day 3, resulted in a significantly shorter ICU LOS and a higher incidence of hypoglycaemia. There was no significant difference in mortality between the two groups. Additionally, the late PN group experienced lower rates of new infections, shorter durations of mechanical ventilation and RRT, shorter hospital LOS, and lower health care costs. However, there was no significant difference in functional status at hospital discharge.
Study Conclusion	'Late initiation of parenteral nutrition was associated with faster recovery and fewer complications, as compared with early initiation.'

EPaNIC (2011): Casaer MP, Mesotten D, Hermans G, et al. Early versus late parenteral nutrition in critically ill adults. N Engl J Med. 2011;365(6):506–517.

Study Name	EDEN (2012)
Population	Adults with acute lung injury requiring mechanical ventilation
Intervention	Trophic enteral feeding vs full enteral feeding
Primary Outcome/s	• **VFDs at day 28**: No significant difference
Secondary Outcome/s	• **60-Day mortality, Infectious complications**: No significant difference • **Gastrointestinal intolerance**: Significantly lower in trophic group (more vomiting, elevated gastric residual volumes, and more constipation in full feeding group)
Viva Summary	In a study involving adults with acute lung injury requiring mechanical ventilation, the comparison between trophic enteral feeding and full enteral feeding revealed no significant difference in the primary outcome of VFDs at day 28. Additionally, there were no significant differences in secondary outcomes, including 60-day mortality and infectious complications. However, gastrointestinal intolerance was significantly lower in the trophic group due to higher incidences of vomiting, higher gastric residual volumes, and constipation observed in the full feeding group.
Study Conclusion	'In patients with acute lung injury, compared with full enteral feeding, a strategy of initial trophic enteral feeding for up to 6 days did not improve ventilator-free days, 60-day mortality, or infectious complications but was associated with less gastrointestinal intolerance.'

EDEN (2012): National Heart, Lung, and Blood Institute Acute Respiratory Distress Syndrome (ARDS) Clinical Trials Network; Rice TW, Wheeler AP, Thompson BT, Steingrub J et al. Initial trophic vs full enteral feeding in patients with acute lung injury: the EDEN randomized trial. JAMA. 2012 Feb 22;307(8):795–803.

Study Name	REDOX (2013)
Population	Critically ill adults with multiorgan failure receiving mechanical ventilation
Intervention	Glutamine +/–antioxidants vs placebo
Primary Outcome/s	• **28-Day mortality**: No significant difference (but trend towards increased mortality with glutamine)
Secondary Outcome/s	• **In-hospital mortality, 6-Month mortality**: Significantly higher with glutamine • Antioxidants had no effect on 28-day mortality or other secondary endpoints
Viva Summary	In a study involving critically ill adults with multiorgan failure who were on mechanical ventilation, administering glutamine with or without antioxidants versus placebo did not result in a significant difference in 28-day mortality, though there was a trend towards increased mortality with glutamine. When assessing secondary outcomes, the in-hospital and 6-month mortality rates were significantly higher in the group receiving glutamine. Antioxidants did not have any effect on 28-day mortality or other secondary endpoints.
Study Conclusion	'Early provision of glutamine or antioxidants did not improve clinical outcomes, and glutamine was associated with an increase in mortality among critically ill patients with multiorgan failure.'

REDOX (2013): Heyland D, Muscedere J, Wischmeyer PE, et al.; Canadian Critical Care Trials Group. A randomized trial of glutamine and antioxidants in critically ill patients. N Engl J Med. 2013 Apr 18;368(16):1489–1497.

Study Name	CALORIES (2014)
Population	Critically ill patients in ICU
Intervention	Parenteral nutrition (PN) via dedicated CVC lumen vs enteral nutrition (EN) via NG/NJ tube
Primary Outcome/s	• **30-Day all-cause mortality**: No significant difference
Secondary Outcome/s	• **Episodes of clinically significant hypoglycaemia, Vomiting**: Significantly lower with PN • **Serious hypoglycaemia, Duration of organ support, Complications, LOS**: No significant difference
Viva Summary	In a study involving critically ill patients in the ICU, the comparison between PN delivered through a dedicated CVC lumen and EN through NG/NJ tube produced no significant difference in 30-day all-cause mortality. However, PN led to significantly fewer episodes of clinically significant hypoglycaemia and vomiting compared to EN, while there were no significant differences in serious hypoglycaemia, duration of organ support, complications, or LOS.
Study Conclusion	'We found no significant difference in 30-day mortality associated with the route of delivery of early nutritional support in critically ill adults.'

CALORIES (2014): Harvey SE, Parrott F, Harrison DA, et al. Trial of the route of early nutritional support in critically ill adults. N Engl J Med. 2014;371(18):1673–1684.

Study Name	PermiT (2015)
Population	Critically ill adults
Intervention	Permissive underfeeding (40–60% requirement) vs standard feeding while maintaining similar protein intake for up to 14 days
Primary Outcome/s	• **90-Day mortality**: No significant difference
Secondary Outcome/s	A number of other secondary outcomes, including mortality at other time frames, adverse effects, feeding intolerance, diarrhoea, rate of infections, and ICU/hospital LOS, showed no significant differences between groups.
Viva Summary	In a study involving critically ill adults, a comparison was made between permissive underfeeding (providing 40–60% of caloric requirement) and standard feeding, while maintaining similar protein intake for up to 14 days. The primary outcome, 90-day mortality, was not significantly different between the two groups. Additionally, various secondary outcomes, such as mortality at different time points, adverse effects, feeding intolerance, diarrhoea, infection rates, and ICU or hospital LOS, were not significantly different between the groups.
Study Conclusion	'Enteral feeding to deliver a moderate amount of nonprotein calories to critically ill adults was not associated with lower mortality than that associated with planned delivery of a full amount of nonprotein calories.'

PermiT (2005): Arabi YM, Aldawood AS, Haddad SH, et al. Permissive underfeeding or standard enteral feeding in critically ill adults. N Engl J Med. 2015; 372(25):2398–2408.

Study Name	EFFORT Protein (2023)
Population	Critically ill adults being mechanically ventilated
Intervention	High protein dose (≥2.2 g/kg per day) vs standard protein dose (≤1.2 g/kg per day)
Primary Outcome/s	• **Incidence of alive hospital discharge by 60 days**: No significant difference
Secondary Outcome/s	• **60-Day mortality, Hospital mortality, Duration of mechanical ventilation, ICU/Hospital LOS**: No significant difference • Subgroup analysis showed that high-dose protein had a worse outcome in patients with concomitant AKI or high SOFA scores
Viva Summary	In a study involving critically ill adults on mechanical ventilation, a comparison was made between the effects of a high protein dose (≥2.2 g/kg per day) and a standard protein dose (≤1.2 g/kg per day). The primary outcome, the incidence of alive hospital discharge by 60 days, showed no significant difference between the two groups. Secondary outcomes, including 60-day mortality, hospital mortality, duration of mechanical ventilation, and ICU/hospital LOS, also did not differ significantly between the high-dose and standard-dose protein groups. However, a subgroup analysis indicated that patients with concomitant AKI or high SOFA scores experienced worse outcomes when receiving the high-dose protein regimen.
Study Conclusion	'Delivery of higher doses of protein to mechanically ventilated critically ill patients did not improve the time-to-discharge-alive from hospital and might have worsened outcomes for patients with acute kidney injury and high organ failure scores.'

EFFORT Protein (2023): Heyland DK, Patel J, Compher C, et al. The effect of higher protein dosing in critically ill patients with high nutritional risk (EFFORT Protein): an international, multicentre, pragmatic, registry-based randomised trial. Lancet. 2023 Feb 18;401(10376):568–576.

STRESS ULCER PROPHYLAXIS

Study Name	SUP-ICU (2018)
Population	ICU patients at risk of GI bleeding
Intervention	Pantoprazole 40 mg IV daily vs placebo
Primary Outcome/s	• **90-Day mortality**: No significant difference
Secondary Outcome/s	• **Clinically important GI bleeding**: Significantly lower in pantoprazole group • **Clinically important events**: No significant difference
Viva Summary	In a study comparing the use of pantoprazole 40 mg IV daily to a placebo in ICU patients at risk of GI bleeding, 90-day mortality was not significantly different between the two groups. However, the secondary outcome of clinically important GI bleeding was significantly lower in the pantoprazole group, while there was no significant difference in clinically important events between the two groups.
Study Conclusion	'Among adult patients in the ICU who were at risk for gastrointestinal bleeding, mortality at 90 days and the number of clinically important events were similar in those assigned to pantoprazole and those assigned to placebo.'

SUP-ICU (2018): Krag M, Marker S, Perner A, et al. Pantoprazole in patients at risk for gastrointestinal bleeding in the ICU. N Engl J Med. 2018;379(23): 2199–2208.

LIVER DISEASE

Study Name	Sort et al. (1999)
Population	Cirrhosis and spontaneous bacterial peritonitis (SBP)
Intervention	Cefotaxime + albumin vs cefotaxime alone
Primary Outcome/s	• **Renal impairment**: Significantly lower with combination therapy
Secondary Outcome/s	• **In-hospital mortality, 3-Month mortality**: Significantly lower with combination therapy
Viva Summary	In a study comparing the treatment of cirrhosis-related SBP, the intervention involving cefotaxime combined with albumin was associated with significantly lower rates of renal impairment compared to treatment with cefotaxime alone. Additionally, the combination therapy resulted in significantly lower in-hospital mortality and 3-month mortality.
Study Conclusion	'In patients with cirrhosis and spontaneous bacterial peritonitis, treatment with intravenous albumin in addition to an antibiotic reduces the incidence of renal impairment and death in comparison with treatment with an antibiotic alone.'

Sort P, Navasa M, Arroyo V, et al. Effect of intravenous albumin on renal impairment and mortality in patients with cirrhosis and spontaneous bacterial peritonitis. N Engl J Med. 1999;341(6):403–409.

Study Name	STOPAH (2015)
Population	Severe alcoholic hepatitis
Intervention	Four groups: Prednisolone vs pentoxifylline vs prednisolone + pentoxifylline vs placebo for 28 days
Primary Outcome/s	• **28-Day mortality**: No significant difference between any individual group • Multivariate analysis of the primary outcome demonstrated a potential benefit with prednisolone at 28 days, but this was not demonstrated to persist to 90 days or 1 year
Secondary Outcome/s	• **90-Day mortality or liver transplant, 1-Year mortality or liver transplant**: No significant difference • **Rate of serious infections**: Significantly greater in prednisolone groups
Viva Summary	In a study involving patients with severe alcoholic hepatitis, four different treatment groups were compared: prednisolone only, pentoxifylline only, prednisolone + pentoxifylline, and placebo only over a 28-day period. The primary outcome of 28-day mortality was not significantly different between any of the treatment groups. However, a multivariate analysis suggested a potential benefit with prednisolone at 28 days, although this benefit did not persist at 90 days or 1 year. Secondary outcomes, including 90-day mortality or liver transplant and 1-year mortality or liver transplant, also did not differ significantly among the groups. Notably, the prednisolone groups had a significantly higher rate of serious infections compared to the other groups.
Study Conclusion	'Pentoxifylline did not improve survival in patients with alcoholic hepatitis. Prednisolone was associated with a reduction in 28-day mortality that did not reach significance and with no improvement in outcomes at 90 days or 1 year.'

STOPAH (2015): Thursz MR, Richardson P, Allison M, et al. Prednisolone or pentoxifylline for alcoholic hepatitis. N Engl J Med. 2015;372(17): 1619–1628.

Study Name	Pettie et al. (2019)
Population	Paracetamol overdose
Intervention	12-Hour NAC regimen (SNAP) vs 21-hour NAC protocol
Primary Outcome/s	• **Hepatotoxicity**: No significant difference
Secondary Outcome/s	• **Antihistamine treatment for NAC anaphylactoid reaction**: Significantly lower in SNAP group
Viva Summary	In a study comparing two treatments for paracetamol overdose, the use of a 12-hour NAC regimen (SNAP) was found to have no significant difference in hepatotoxicity when compared to a 21-hour NAC protocol. However, the SNAP group experienced significantly fewer anaphylactoid reactions requiring antihistamine treatment compared to the 21-hour protocol group.
Study Conclusion	'In clinical use the SNAP regimen has similar efficacy as standard therapy for preventing liver injury and produces fewer adverse reactions.'

Pettie JM, Caparrotta TM, Hunter RW, et al. Safety and efficacy of the snap 12-hour acetylcysteine regimen for the treatment of paracetamol overdose. EClinicalMedicine. 2019;11:11–17.

UPPER GI BLEEDING

Study Name	Villanueva et al. (2013)
Population	Severe acute UGIB
Intervention	Restrictive transfusion strategy (threshold 70 g/l) vs liberal transfusion strategy (threshold 90 g/l)
Primary Outcome/s	• **45-Day mortality**: Significantly lower with restrictive transfusion
Secondary Outcome/s	• **Further bleeding, In-hospital complications**: Significantly lower with restrictive transfusion • **Portal pressure gradient within 5 days**: Significantly increased in liberal transfusion group
Viva Summary	In a study comparing restrictive transfusion (threshold 70 g/l) with liberal transfusion (threshold 90 g/l) strategies for patients with severe acute UGI bleeding, the primary outcome of 45-day mortality was significantly lower in the restrictive transfusion group. Additionally, the secondary outcomes of further bleeding and in-hospital complications were also significantly lower in the restrictive transfusion group, while the portal pressure gradient within 5 days was significantly increased in the liberal transfusion group.
Study Conclusion	'As compared with a liberal transfusion strategy, a restrictive strategy significantly improved outcomes in patients with acute upper gastrointestinal bleeding.'

Villanueva C, Colomo A, Bosch A, et al. Transfusion strategies for acute upper gastrointestinal bleeding. N Engl J Med. 2013;368(1):11–21.

Study Name	Escorsell et al. (2016)
Population	Patients with cirrhosis and oesophageal variceal bleeding refractory to medical and endoscopic treatment
Intervention	Oesophageal covered metal stent vs balloon tamponade
Primary Outcome/s	• **Composite of survival at day 15, Control of bleeding, and absence of serious adverse events**: Significantly higher with metal stent
Secondary Outcome/s	• **Success of therapy, Control of bleeding**: Significantly higher in stent group • **6-Week survival, Transfusion requirements, Serious adverse events**: No significant difference
Viva Summary	In a study involving patients with cirrhosis and oesophageal variceal bleeding refractory to medical and endoscopic treatment, the primary composite outcome of survival at day 15, control of bleeding, and absence of serious adverse events was significantly better in the oesophageal covered metal stent group compared to balloon tamponade. Additionally, secondary outcomes, including the success of therapy and control of bleeding, were also notably higher in the stent group, while there were no significant differences in 6-week survival, transfusion requirements, or serious adverse events between the two interventions.
Study Conclusion	'Esophageal stents have greater efficacy with less SAEs than balloon tamponade in the control of EVB in treatment failures. Our findings favor the use of esophageal stents in patients with EVB uncontrolled with medical and endoscopic treatment.'

Escorsell À, Pavel O, Cárdenas A, et al. Esophageal balloon tamponade versus esophageal stent in controlling acute refractory variceal bleeding: a multicenter randomized, controlled trial. Hepatology. 2016;63(6):1957–1967.

Study Name	HALT-IT (2020)
Population	Patients with significant GI bleeding
Intervention	Tranexamic acid (TXA) 1-g followed by infusion of 3-g over 24 hours vs placebo
Primary Outcome/s	• **Death due to bleeding within 5 days**: No significant difference
Secondary Outcome/s	• **VTE**: Significantly higher in TXA group • **24-Hour/28-Day mortality, Rebleeding, Interventions required, Transfusions required**: No significant difference
Viva Summary	In a study involving patients with significant gastrointestinal bleeding, the use of TXA at a dosage of 1-g followed by a 3-g over 24-hour infusion, compared to placebo, did not result in a significant difference in death due to bleeding within 5 days. However, the TXA group experienced a significantly higher incidence of VTE as a secondary outcome. Other secondary outcomes, such as 24-hour/28-day mortality, rebleeding, interventions required, and transfusions required, were not significantly different.
Study Conclusion	'We found that tranexamic acid did not reduce death from gastrointestinal bleeding. On the basis of our results, tranexamic acid should not be used for the treatment of gastrointestinal bleeding outside the context of a randomised trial.'

HALT-IT (2020): The HALT-IT Trial Collaborators. Effects of a high-dose 24h infusion of tranexamic acid on death and thromboembolic events in patients with acute gastrointestinal bleeding (HALT-IT): an international randomised, double-blind, placebo- controlled trial. Lancet. 2020;395(10241): 1927–1936.

SELECTIVE DECONTAMINATION OF THE DIGESTIVE TRACT

Study Name	SuDDICU (2022)
Population	Mechanically ventilated adults in ICUs in Australia
Intervention	Selective decontamination of the digestive tract (SDD) vs standard care
Primary Outcome/s	• **In-hospital 90-day mortality**: No significant difference
Secondary Outcome/s	• **ICU mortality, Days alive and free from mechanical ventilation, Incidence of new *Clostridium difficile* infection, Adverse medication events**: No significant difference • **Antibiotic-resistant organisms, New positive blood cultures**: Significantly lower in SDD group • In ecological assessment, SDD was found to be as effective as standard care in preventing newly positive blood cultures and *C. difficile* infections (non-inferior). However, it did not demonstrate the same effectiveness for cultures of antibiotic-resistant organisms
Viva Summary	In Australia, a study compared the use of SDD with standard care for mechanically ventilated adults in ICUs. The primary outcome, which was 90-day in-hospital mortality, did not show a significant difference between the two groups. Secondary outcomes, including ICU mortality, days without mechanical ventilation, the incidence of *C. difficile* infection, and adverse medication events, also did not differ significantly between the groups. However, the incidence of antibiotic-resistant organisms and new positive blood cultures were significantly lower in the SDD group. An ecological assessment found SDD to be non-inferior to standard care in preventing new positive blood cultures and *C. difficile* infections, but it did not demonstrate the same effectiveness for cultures of antibiotic-resistant organisms.

(Continued)

(Continued)

Study Name	SuDDICU (2022)
Study Conclusion	'Among critically ill patients receiving mechanical ventilation, SDD, compared with standard care without SDD, did not significantly reduce in-hospital mortality. However, the confidence interval around the effect estimate includes a clinically important benefit.'

SuDDICU (2022): SuDDICU Investigators for the Australian and New Zealand Intensive Care Society Clinical Trials Group; Myburgh JA, Seppelt IM, Goodman F, et al. Effect of selective decontamination of the digestive tract on hospital mortality in critically ill patients receiving mechanical ventilation: a randomized clinical trial. JAMA. 2022 Nov 15;328(19):1911–1921.

GLUCOSE MANAGEMENT

Study Name	NICE-SUGAR (2009)
Population	Critically unwell adults
Intervention	Intensive glucose control (target 4.5–6 mmol/l) vs conventional glucose control (<10 mmol/l)
Primary Outcome/s	• **90-Day all-cause mortality**: Significantly higher in intensive glucose control group
Secondary Outcome/s	• **Severe hypoglycaemia**: Significantly higher in intensive glucose control group • **28-Day mortality, LOS, Organ support**: No significant difference
Viva Summary	In a study involving critically ill adults, two approaches to glucose control were compared: intensive control with a target range of 4.5–6 mmol/l and conventional control with a target of <10 mmol/l. Ninety-day all-cause mortality was significantly higher in the intensive glucose control group, while the secondary outcome of severe hypoglycaemia was also significantly increased in the intensive glucose control group. However, there were no significant differences in 28-day mortality, hospital LOS, or the need for organ support between the two groups.
Study Conclusion	'In this large, international, randomized trial, we found that intensive glucose control increased mortality among adults in the ICU: a blood glucose target of 10 mmol/l or less resulted in lower mortality than did a target of 5–6 mmol/l.'

NICE-SUGAR (2009): The NICE-SUGAR Study Investigators. Intensive versus conventional glucose control in critically ill patients. N Engl J Med. 2009;360(13):1283–1297.

ACUTE PANCREATITIS

Study Name	de-Madaria et al. (2022)
Population	Adults with acute pancreatitis
Intervention	Aggressive fluid resuscitation (bolus 20 ml/kg, then 3 ml/kg/hr infusion) vs moderate fluid resuscitation (bolus 10 ml/kg in hypovolemia then 1.5 ml/kg/hr infusion)
Primary Outcome/s	• **Occurrence of moderately severe or severe pancreatitis**: No significant difference
Secondary Outcome/s	• **Severe pancreatitis, Local complications, ICU admission, Persistent organ failure, Persistent SIRS, Mortality**: No significant difference • **Fluid overload**: Significantly higher in aggressive fluid group leading to early trial termination
Viva Summary	In a study comparing aggressive fluid resuscitation (20 ml/kg bolus followed by 3 ml/kg/hr) with moderate fluid resuscitation (10 ml/kg bolus in hypovolemia then 1.5 ml/kg/hr) for adults with acute pancreatitis, there was no significant difference in the occurrence of moderately severe or severe pancreatitis as the primary outcome. Secondary outcomes, including local complications, ICU admission, persistent organ failure, persistent SIRS, and mortality, also showed no significant differences between the two groups. However, the aggressive fluid group had a significantly higher incidence of fluid overload, which led to the early termination of the trial.
Study Conclusion	'In this randomized trial involving patients with acute pancreatitis, early aggressive fluid resuscitation resulted in a higher incidence of fluid overload without improvement in clinical outcomes.'

de-Madaria E, Buxbaum JL, Maisonneuve P, et al.; ERICA Consortium. Aggressive or moderate fluid resuscitation in acute pancreatitis. N Engl J Med. 2022 Sep 15;387(11):989–1000.

SUMMARY

1. **TICACOS (2011):** In a study involving critically ill adult patients requiring mechanical ventilation for more than 3 days, two nutritional support approaches were compared: one guided by daily REE measurements and the other based on a fixed weight-based regimen of 25 kcal/kg/day. The primary outcome, hospital mortality, was not significantly different between the two groups. However, secondary outcome analysis showed that the REE-guided group received more energy, had a higher rate of parenteral nutrition in the first 3 days, and experienced longer durations of ventilation and ICU LOS compared to the weight-based regimen group.

2. **OMEGA (2011):** In a study involving adults with acute lung injury requiring mechanical ventilation, the effects of enteral supplementation of n-3 fatty acids, γ-linolenic acids, and antioxidants were compared with an isocaloric control group. The intervention group had significantly fewer VFDs to day 28, experienced significantly lower non-pulmonary organ failure–free days and ICU-free days, and also had more days with diarrhoea. Additionally, there was a higher 60-day mortality rate in the intervention group, although the statistical significance was borderline. The study was halted prematurely due to concerns about potential harm or futility.

3. **EPaNIC (2011):** In a study comparing the timing of PN in critically ill adults, it was found that administering PN on day 8, rather than on day 3, resulted in a significantly shorter ICU LOS and a higher incidence of hypoglycaemia. There was no significant difference in mortality between the two groups. Additionally, the late PN group experienced lower rates of new infections, shorter durations of mechanical ventilation and RRT, shorter hospital LOS, and lower health care costs. However, there was no significant difference in functional status at hospital discharge.

4. **EDEN (2012):** In a study involving adults with acute lung injury requiring mechanical ventilation, the comparison between trophic enteral feeding and full enteral feeding revealed no significant difference in the primary outcome of VFDs at day 28. Additionally, there were no significant differences in secondary outcomes,

including 60-day mortality and infectious complications. However, gastrointestinal intolerance was significantly lower in the trophic group due to higher incidences of vomiting, higher gastric residual volumes, and constipation observed in the full feeding group.

5. **REDOX (2013):** In a study involving critically ill adults with multiorgan failure who were on mechanical ventilation, administering glutamine with or without antioxidants versus placebo did not result in a significant difference in 28-day mortality, though there was a trend towards increased mortality with glutamine. When assessing secondary outcomes, the in-hospital and 6-month mortality rates were significantly higher in the group receiving glutamine. Antioxidants did not have any effect on 28-day mortality or other secondary endpoints.

6. **CALORIES (2014):** In a study involving critically ill patients in the ICU, the comparison between PN delivered through a dedicated CVC lumen and EN through NG/NJ tube produced no significant difference in 30-day all-cause mortality. However, PN led to significantly fewer episodes of clinically significant hypoglycaemia and vomiting compared to EN, while there were no significant differences in serious hypoglycaemia, duration of organ support, complications, or LOS.

7. **PermiT (2015):** In a study involving critically ill adults, a comparison was made between permissive underfeeding (providing 40–60% of caloric requirement) and standard feeding, while maintaining similar protein intake for up to 14 days. The primary outcome, 90-day mortality, was not significantly different between the two groups. Additionally, various secondary outcomes, such as mortality at different time points, adverse effects, feeding intolerance, diarrhoea, infection rates, and ICU or hospital LOS, were not significantly different between the groups.

8. **EFFORT Protein (2023):** In a study involving critically ill adults on mechanical ventilation, a comparison was made between the effects of a high protein dose (≥ 2.2 g/kg per day) and a standard protein dose (≤ 1.2 g/kg per day). The primary outcome, the incidence of alive hospital discharge by 60 days, showed no significant difference between the two groups. Secondary outcomes, including 60-day mortality, hospital mortality, duration of mechanical ventilation, and ICU/hospital LOS, also did not differ significantly between the

high-dose and standard-dose protein groups. However, a subgroup analysis indicated that patients with concomitant AKI or high SOFA scores experienced worse outcomes when receiving the high-dose protein regimen.

9. **SUP-ICU (2018):** In a study comparing the use of pantoprazole 40 mg IV daily to a placebo in ICU patients at risk of GI bleeding, 90-day mortality was not significantly different between the two groups. However, the secondary outcome of clinically important GI bleeding was significantly lower in the pantoprazole group, while there was no significant difference in clinically important events between the two groups.

10. **Sort et al. (1999):** In a study comparing the treatment of cirrhosis-related SBP, the intervention involving cefotaxime combined with albumin was associated with significantly lower rates of renal impairment compared to treatment with cefotaxime alone. Additionally, the combination therapy resulted in significantly lower in-hospital mortality and 3-month mortality.

11. **STOPAH (2015):** In a study involving patients with severe alcoholic hepatitis, four different treatment groups were compared: prednisolone only, pentoxifylline only, prednisolone + pentoxifylline, and placebo only over a 28-day period. The primary outcome of 28-day mortality was not significantly different between any of the treatment groups. However, a multivariate analysis suggested a potential benefit with prednisolone at 28 days, although this benefit did not persist at 90 days or 1 year. Secondary outcomes, including 90-day mortality or liver transplant and 1-year mortality of liver transplant, also did not differ significantly among the groups. Notably, the prednisolone groups had a significantly higher rate of serious infections compared to the other groups.

12. **Pettie et al. (2019):** In a study comparing two treatments for paracetamol overdose, the use of a 12-hour NAC regimen (SNAP) was found to have no significant difference in hepatotoxicity when compared to a 21-hour NAC protocol. However, the SNAP group experienced significantly fewer anaphylactoid reactions requiring antihistamine treatment compared to the 21-hour protocol group.

13. **Villanueva et al. (2013):** In a study comparing restrictive transfusion (threshold 70 g/l) with liberal transfusion (threshold 90 g/l) strategies for patients with severe acute UGI bleeding,

the primary outcome of 45-day mortality was significantly lower in the restrictive transfusion group. Additionally, the secondary outcomes of further bleeding and in-hospital complications were also significantly lower in the restrictive transfusion group, while the portal pressure gradient within 5 days was significantly increased in the liberal transfusion group.

14. **Escorsell et al. (2016):** In a study involving patients with cirrhosis and oesophageal variceal bleeding refractory to medical and endoscopic treatment, the primary composite outcome of survival at day 15, control of bleeding, and absence of serious adverse events was significantly better in the oesophageal covered metal stent group compared to balloon tamponade. Additionally, secondary outcomes, including the success of therapy and control of bleeding, were also notably higher in the stent group, while there were no significant differences in 6-week survival, transfusion requirements, or serious adverse events between the two interventions.

15. **HALT-IT (2020):** In a study involving patients with significant gastrointestinal bleeding, the use of TXA at a dosage of 1 g followed by a 3 g over 24-hour infusion, compared to placebo, did not result in a significant difference in death due to bleeding within 5 days. However, the TXA group experienced a significantly higher incidence of VTE as a secondary outcome. Other secondary outcomes, such as 24-hour/28-day mortality, rebleeding, interventions required, and transfusions required, were not significantly different.

16. **SuDDICU (2022):** In Australia, a study compared the use of SDD with standard care for mechanically ventilated adults in ICUs. The primary outcome, which was 90-day in-hospital mortality, did not show a significant difference between the two groups. Secondary outcomes, including ICU mortality, days without mechanical ventilation, the incidence of *C. difficile* infection, and adverse medication events, also did not differ significantly between the groups. However, the incidence of antibiotic-resistant organisms and new positive blood cultures were significantly lower in the SDD group. An ecological assessment found SDD to be non-inferior to standard care in preventing new positive blood cultures and *C. difficile* infections, but it did not demonstrate the same effectiveness for cultures of antibiotic-resistant organisms.

17. **NICE-SUGAR (2009):** In a study involving critically ill adults, two approaches to glucose control were compared: intensive control with a target range of 4.5–6 mmol/l and conventional control with a target of <10 mmol/l. Ninety-day all-cause mortality was significantly higher in the intensive glucose control group, while the secondary outcome of severe hypoglycaemia was also significantly increased in the intensive glucose control group. However, there were no significant differences in 28-day mortality, hospital LOS, or the need for organ support between the two groups.

18. **de-Madaria et al. (2022):** In a study comparing aggressive fluid resuscitation (20 ml/kg bolus followed by 3 ml/kg/hr) with moderate fluid resuscitation (10 ml/kg bolus in hypovolemia then 1.5 ml/kg/hr) for adults with acute pancreatitis, there was no significant difference in the occurrence of moderately severe or severe pancreatitis as the primary outcome. Secondary outcomes, including local complications, ICU admission, persistent organ failure, persistent SIRS, and mortality, also showed no significant differences between the two groups. However, the aggressive fluid group had a significantly higher incidence of fluid overload, which led to the early termination of the trial.

ACUTE KIDNEY INJURY/RENAL REPLACEMENT THERAPY (RRT)

Study Name	ATN (2008)
Population	Critically ill patients with AKI consistent with acute tubular necrosis (ATN)
Intervention	Intensive vs conventional RRT (IHD, CVVHDF, or SLEDD, determined by SOFA)
Primary Outcome/s	• **60-Day all-cause mortality**: No significant difference
Secondary Outcome/s	• **In-hospital mortality, Recovery of renal function, Organ failure–free days**: No significant difference
Viva Summary	In a study involving critically ill patients with ATN, intensive RRT was compared with conventional RRT. The primary outcome of 60-day all-cause mortality was not significantly different between the two groups, and secondary outcomes, including in-hospital mortality, recovery of renal function, and organ failure–free days were also not significantly different.
Study Conclusion	'Intensive renal support in critically ill patients with acute kidney injury did not decrease mortality, improve recovery of kidney function, or reduce the rate of nonrenal organ failure as compared with less-intensive therapy involving a defined dose of intermittent hemodialysis three times per week and continuous renal-replacement therapy at 20 ml per kilogram per hour.'

ATN (2008): VA/NIH Acute Renal Failure Trial Network. Intensity of renal support in critically ill patients with acute kidney injury. N Engl J Med. 2008;359(1):7–20.

DOI: 10.1201/9781003468738-5

Study Name	RENAL (2009)
Population	Critically ill adults with AKI requiring RRT
Intervention	High-intensity CVVHDF (40 ml/kg/h) vs standard-intensity CVVHDF (25 ml/kg/h)
Primary Outcome/s	• **90-Day all-cause mortality**: No significant difference
Secondary Outcome/s	• **Duration of RRT, 28-Day mortality, In-hospital mortality**: No significant difference • **Hypophosphataemia**: Increased incidence in high-intensity group
Viva Summary	In a study involving critically ill adults with AKI requiring RRT, high-intensity CVVHDF at 40 ml/kg/h was compared to standard-intensity CVVHDF at 25 ml/kg/h. There was no significant difference in 90-day all-cause mortality between the two groups. Similarly, secondary outcomes including the duration of RRT, 28-day mortality, and in-hospital mortality were not significantly different. However, the high-intensity group did experience an increased incidence of hypophosphataemia.
Study Conclusion	'In critically ill patients with acute kidney injury, treatment with higher-intensity continuous renal-replacement therapy did not reduce mortality at 90 days.'

RENAL (2009): The RENAL Replacement Therapy Study Investigators. Intensity of continuous renal-replacement therapy in critically ill patients. N Engl J Med. 2009;361(17):1627–1638.

Study Name	CARRESS-HF (2012)
Population	Acute decompensated heart failure and cardiorenal syndrome
Intervention	Slow Continuous Ultrafiltration (SCUF) vs medical management
Primary Outcome/s	• **Change in serum creatinine and weight at day 4**: No significant difference in weight but worsening of serum creatinine in the SCUF group (contradicting the goal of renal improvement)
Secondary Outcome/s	• **60-Day all-cause mortality, Weight loss, Renal improvement**: No significant difference • **Adverse events**: Significantly higher in SCUF group (increased incidence of CHF, renal failure, bleeding complications, and catheter-related complications) • Trial terminated early due to futility and an excess of adverse events in the SCUF arm
Viva Summary	In a study comparing SCUF with medical management in patients with acute decompensated heart failure and cardiorenal syndrome, there was no significant difference in weight change at day 4. However, there was a significant rise in serum creatinine in the SCUF group, contrary to the goal of renal improvement. Secondary outcomes, including 60-day all-cause mortality, weight loss, and renal improvement, showed no significant differences between the two groups. Nevertheless, the SCUF group experienced significantly more adverse events, such as increased incidences of CHF, renal failure, bleeding complications, and catheter-related complications. This led to the early termination of the trial due to futility and the excessive number of adverse events in the SCUF arm.
Study Conclusion	'In a randomized trial involving patients hospitalized for acute decompensated heart failure, worsened renal function, and persistent congestion, the use of a stepped pharmacologic-therapy algorithm was superior to a strategy of ultrafiltration for the preservation of renal function at 96 hours, with a similar amount of weight loss with the two approaches. Ultrafiltration was associated with a higher rate of adverse events.'

CARRESS-HF (2012): Bart BA, Goldsmith SR, Lee KL, et al. Ultrafiltration in decompensated heart failure with cardiorenal syndrome. N Engl J Med. 2012;367(24):2296–2304.

Study Name	IVOIRE (2013)
Population	Critically ill patients with septic shock and AKI for <24 hours
Intervention	High-volume haemofiltration (HVHF) (70 ml/kg/h) vs standard-volume haemofiltration (SVHF) (35 ml/kg/h) for 96 hours
Primary Outcome/s	• **28-Day mortality**: No significant difference
Secondary Outcome/s	• There were no statistically significant differences in any of the secondary endpoints between treatment groups • The trial was halted due to low patient enrolment and resource constraints
Viva Summary	In a study conducted on critically ill patients with septic shock and AKI for less than 24 hours, the effects of HVHF at a rate of 70 ml/kg/h were compared to SVHF at a rate of 35 ml/kg/h over a 96-hour period. The primary outcome of 28-day mortality rate was not significantly different between the two groups. Additionally, there were no statistically significant variations in any of the secondary endpoints. The trial was stopped due to limited patient enrolment and resource constraints.
Study Conclusion	'In the IVOIRE trial, there was no evidence that HVHF at 70 mL/kg/h, when compared with contemporary SVHF at 35 mL/kg/h, leads to a reduction of 28-day mortality or contributes to early improvements in haemodynamic profile or organ function. HVHF, as applied in this trial, cannot be recommended for treatment of septic shock complicated by AKI.'

IVOIRE (2013): Joannes-Boyau O, Honoré PM, Perez P, et al. High-volume versus standard-volume haemofiltration for septic shock patients with acute kidney injury (IVOIRE study): a multicentre randomized controlled trial. Intensive Care Med. 2013;39(9):1535–1546.

Study Name	AKIKI (2016)
Population	Critically ill patients with stage 3 AKI but no life-threatening complication directly related to renal failure
Intervention	Early RRT <6 hours vs delayed RRT using conventional criteria, e.g. hyperkalaemia
Primary Outcome/s	• **60-Day mortality**: No significant difference
Secondary Outcome/s	• **8-Day mortality, ICU/Hospital LOS, RRT dependency**: No significant difference • **Number receiving RRT, Catheter-related bloodstream infections (CRBSIs)**: Significantly higher in early group
Viva Summary	In a study involving critically ill patients diagnosed with stage 3 AKI without immediate life-threatening complications related to renal failure, a comparison was made between those who received early RRT within 6 hours and those who underwent delayed RRT based on traditional criteria like hyperkalaemia. The primary outcome, 60-day mortality, was not significantly different between the two groups. Similarly, secondary outcomes, including 8-day mortality, ICU/hospital LOS, and RRT dependency, were not significantly different. However, the early RRT group had a significantly higher number of patients receiving RRT and experienced more CRBSIs compared to the delayed group.
Study Conclusion	'In a trial involving critically ill patients with severe acute kidney injury, we found no significant difference with regard to mortality between an early and a delayed strategy for the initiation of renal-replacement therapy. A delayed strategy averted the need for renal-replacement therapy in an appreciable number of patients.'

AKIKI (2016): Gaudry S, Hajage D, Schortgen F, et al. Initiation strategies for renal-replacement therapy in the intensive care unit. N Engl J Med. 2016;375(2):122–133.

Study Name	ELAIN (2016)
Population	Critically ill patients with severe AKI (single-centre study with predominantly surgical population)
Intervention	Early RRT (within 8 hours of stage 2 AKI) vs delayed RRT (within 12 hours of stage 3 AKI)
Primary Outcome/s	• **90-Day mortality**: Significantly lower in the early group
Secondary Outcome/s	• **Duration of RRT, Hospital LOS**: Significantly lower in the early RRT group • **Recovery of renal function by day 90**: Significantly higher in the early RRT group • **Requirement for RRT after day 90, Organ dysfunction, ICU LOS**: No significant difference
Viva Summary	In a single-centre study primarily involving surgical patients, a comparison was made between critically ill individuals with severe AKI who received early RRT within 8 hours of reaching stage 2 AKI and those who received delayed RRT within 12 hours of reaching stage 3 AKI. The primary outcome of 90-day mortality was significantly lower in the early RRT group. Additionally, the early RRT group experienced significantly shorter durations of RRT, reduced hospital LOS, and a higher rate of renal function recovery by day 90, while no significant differences were observed in the need for RRT after day 90, organ dysfunction, or ICU LOS.
Study Conclusion	'Among critically ill patients with AKI, early RRT compared with delayed initiation of RRT reduced mortality over the first 90 days. Further multicenter trials of this intervention are warranted.'

ELAIN (2016): Zarbock A, Kellum JA, Schmidt C, et al. Effect of early vs delayed initiation of renal replacement therapy on mortality in critically ill patients with acute kidney injury: the ELAIN randomized clinical trial. JAMA. 2016;315(20):2190–2199.

Study Name	BICAR-ICU (2018)
Population	Critically ill patients with severe metabolic acidosis (pH ≤7.20)
Intervention	4.25% sodium bicarbonate infusion to maintain pH >7.3 vs no sodium bicarbonate
Primary Outcome/s	• **Composite 28-day mortality and ≥1 organ failure at 7 days**: No significant difference • Sodium bicarbonate showed a significant advantage over the control group in the subgroup of patients with AKI stage 2–3, with improvements in the primary composite outcome, day 28 mortality, and ≥1 organ failures at day 7
Secondary Outcome/s	• **RRT use**: Significantly lower in the bicarbonate group • **RRT-free days, Time to initiation of RRT**: Significantly higher in the bicarbonate group • **ICU LOS, Dependence on dialysis at ICU discharge**: No significant difference • Metabolic alkalosis, hypernatraemia, and hypocalcaemia were more frequent in the bicarbonate group, but no life-threatening complications were reported
Viva Summary	In a study involving critically ill patients with severe metabolic acidosis (pH ≤7.20), the use of a 4.25% sodium bicarbonate infusion to maintain a pH >7.3 compared to no sodium bicarbonate did not show a significant difference in the primary composite outcome of 28-day mortality and presence of at least one organ failure at 7 days. However, in patients with AKI stage 2–3, sodium bicarbonate demonstrated a significant advantage, with improvements in the primary composite outcome, day 28 mortality, and ≥1 organ failures at day 7. Additionally, the bicarbonate group had significantly lower use of RRT, more RRT-free days, and delayed initiation of RRT. There were higher incidences of metabolic alkalosis, hypernatraemia, and hypocalcaemia in the bicarbonate group, but no life-threatening complications were reported. Other outcomes such as ICU LOS and dependence on dialysis at ICU discharge were not significantly different.

(Continued)

(Continued)

Study Name	BICAR-ICU (2018)
Study Conclusion	'In patients with severe metabolic acidaemia, sodium bicarbonate had no effect on the primary composite outcome. However, sodium bicarbonate decreased the primary composite outcome and day 28 mortality in the a-priori defined stratum of patients with acute kidney injury.'

BICAR-ICU (2018): Jaber S, Paugam C, Futier E, et al. Sodium bicarbonate therapy for patients with severe metabolic acidaemia in the intensive care unit (BICAR-ICU): a multicentre, open-label, randomised controlled, phase 3 trial. Lancet. 2018;392(10141):31–40.

Study Name	STARRT-AKI (2020)
Population	Critically ill patients with severe AKI
Intervention	Accelerated RRT (<12 hours of randomisation) vs standard care (classical indications or AKI >72 hours)
Primary Outcome/s	• **90-Day all-cause mortality**: No significant difference
Secondary Outcome/s	• **Composite of death/dependence, MAKE, Sustained reduction in kidney function, ICU mortality at 28 days, Hospital LOS**: No significant difference • **RRT dependence at 90 days, Incidence of adverse events**: Significantly higher in accelerated RRT group
Viva Summary	In a study involving critically ill patients with severe AKI, two interventions were compared: accelerated RRT administered within 12 hours of randomisation and standard care based on classical indications or AKI lasting over 72 hours. Ninety-day all-cause mortality did not significantly differ between the two groups. Additionally, there were no significant differences in various secondary outcomes, including a composite of death or dependence, major adverse kidney events, sustained reduction in kidney function, 28-day ICU mortality, and hospital LOS. However, the accelerated RRT group had a significantly higher incidence of RRT dependence at 90 days and incidence of adverse events compared to the standard care group.
Study Conclusion	'Among critically ill patients with acute kidney injury, an accelerated renal-replacement strategy was not associated with a lower risk of death at 90 days than a standard strategy.'

STARRT-AKI (2020): The STARRT-AKI Investigators for the Canadian Critical Care Trials Group, the Australian and New Zealand Intensive Care Society Clinical Trials Group, the United Kingdom Critical Care Research Group, the Canadian Nephrology Trials Network, and the Irish Critical Care Trials Group. Timing of initiation of renal-replacement therapy in acute kidney injury. N Engl J Med. 2020;383(3):240–251.

Study Name	Zarbock et al. (2020)
Population	Critically ill patients with AKI receiving RRT
Intervention	Regional citrate anticoagulation vs systemic heparin anticoagulation
Primary Outcome/s	• **Filter lifespan**: Significantly higher with regional citrate • **90-Day mortality**: No significant difference
Secondary Outcome/s	• **Bleeding complications**: Significantly lower with regional citrate • **New infections**: Significantly higher with regional citrate
Viva Summary	In a study involving critically ill patients with AKI receiving RRT, a comparison was made between the use of regional citrate anticoagulation and systemic heparin anticoagulation. The regional citrate group had a significantly longer filter lifespan, while there was no significant difference in 90-day mortality between the two groups. Additionally, secondary outcomes indicated that regional citrate was associated with significantly fewer bleeding complications but a higher incidence of new infections compared to systemic heparin anticoagulation.
Study Conclusion	'Among critically ill patients with acute kidney injury receiving continuous kidney replacement therapy, anticoagulation with regional citrate, compared with systemic heparin anticoagulation, resulted in significantly longer filter life span. The trial was terminated early and was therefore underpowered to reach conclusions about the effect of anticoagulation strategy on mortality.'

Zarbock A, Küllmar M, Kindgen-Milles D, et al. Effect of regional citrate anticoagulation vs systemic heparin anticoagulation during continuous kidney replacement therapy on dialysis filter life span and mortality among critical care patients with acute kidney injury: a randomized clinical trial. JAMA. 2020;324(16): 1629–1639.

SUMMARY

1. **ATN (2008):** In a study involving critically ill patients with ATN, intensive RRT was compared with conventional RRT. The primary outcome of 60-day all-cause mortality was not significantly different between the two groups, and secondary outcomes, including in-hospital mortality, recovery of renal function, and organ failure–free days, were also not significantly different.

2. **RENAL (2009):** In a study involving critically ill adults with AKI requiring RRT, high-intensity CVVHDF at 40 ml/kg/h was compared to standard-intensity CVVHDF at 25 ml/kg/h. There was no significant difference in 90-day all-cause mortality between the two groups. Similarly, secondary outcomes including the duration of RRT, 28-day mortality, and in-hospital mortality were not significantly different. However, the high-intensity group did experience an increased incidence of hypophosphataemia.

3. **CARRESS-HF (2012):** In a study comparing SCUF with medical management in patients with acute decompensated heart failure and cardiorenal syndrome, there was no significant difference in weight change at day 4. However, there was a significant rise in serum creatinine in the SCUF group, contrary to the goal of renal improvement. Secondary outcomes, including 60-day all-cause mortality, weight loss, and renal improvement, showed no significant differences between the two groups. Nevertheless, the SCUF group experienced significantly more adverse events, such as increased incidences of CHF, renal failure, bleeding complications, and catheter-related complications. This led to the early termination of the trial due to futility and the excessive number of adverse events in the SCUF arm.

4. **IVOIRE (2013):** In a study conducted on critically ill patients with septic shock and AKI for less than 24 hours, the effects of HVHF at a rate of 70 ml/kg/h were compared to SVHF at a rate of 35 ml/kg/h over a 96-hour period. The primary outcome of 28-day mortality rate was not significantly different between the two groups. Additionally, there were no statistically significant variations in any of the secondary endpoints. The trial was stopped due to limited patient enrolment and resource constraints.

5. **AKIKI (2016):** In a study involving critically ill patients diagnosed with stage 3 AKI without immediate life-threatening complications related to renal failure, a comparison was made between those who received early RRT within 6 hours and those who underwent delayed RRT based on traditional criteria like hyperkalaemia. The primary outcome, 60-day mortality, was not significantly different between the two groups. Similarly, secondary outcomes, including 8-day mortality, ICU/hospital LOS, and RRT dependency, were not significantly different. However, the early RRT group had a significantly higher number of patients receiving RRT and experienced more CRBSIs compared to the delayed group.

6. **ELAIN (2016):** In a single-centre study primarily involving surgical patients, a comparison was made between critically ill individuals with severe AKI who received early RRT within 8 hours of reaching stage 2 AKI and those who received delayed RRT within 12 hours of reaching stage 3 AKI. The primary outcome of 90-day mortality was significantly lower in the early RRT group. Additionally, the early RRT group experienced significantly shorter durations of RRT, reduced hospital LOS, and a higher rate of renal function recovery by day 90, while no significant differences were observed in the need for RRT after day 90, organ dysfunction, or ICU LOS.

7. **BICAR-ICU (2018):** In a study involving critically ill patients with severe metabolic acidosis (pH ≤7.20), the use of a 4.25% sodium bicarbonate infusion to maintain a pH >7.3 compared to no sodium bicarbonate did not show a significant difference in the primary composite outcome of 28-day mortality and presence of at least one organ failure at 7 days. However, in patients with AKI stage 2–3, sodium bicarbonate demonstrated a significant advantage, with improvements in the primary composite outcome, day 28 mortality, and ≥1 organ failures at day 7. Additionally, the bicarbonate group had significantly lower use of RRT, more RRT-free days, and a delayed initiation of RRT. There were higher incidences of metabolic alkalosis, hypernatraemia, and hypocalcaemia in the bicarbonate group, but no life-threatening complications were reported. Other outcomes such as ICU LOS and dependence on dialysis at ICU discharge were not significantly different.

8. **STARRT-AKI (2020):** In a study involving critically ill patients with severe AKI, two interventions were compared: accelerated RRT administered within 12 hours of randomisation and standard care based on classical indications or AKI lasting over 72 hours. Ninety-day all-cause mortality did not significantly differ between the two groups. Additionally, there were no significant differences in various secondary outcomes, including a composite of death or dependence, major adverse kidney events, sustained reduction in kidney function, 28-day ICU mortality, and hospital LOS. However, the accelerated RRT group had a significantly higher incidence of RRT dependence at 90 days and incidence of adverse events compared to the standard care group.

9. **Zarbock et al. (2020):** In a study involving critically ill patients with AKI receiving RRT, a comparison was made between the use of regional citrate anticoagulation and systemic heparin anticoagulation. The regional citrate group had a significantly longer filter lifespan, while there was no significant difference in 90-day mortality between the two groups. Additionally, secondary outcomes indicated that regional citrate was associated with significantly fewer bleeding complications but a higher incidence of new infections compared to systemic heparin anticoagulation.

TRANSFUSION TARGETS

Study Name	TRICC (1999)
Population	Critically ill patients with euvolaemia
Intervention	Restrictive red-cell transfusion threshold (Hb 70 g/l) vs liberal red-cell transfusion threshold (Hb 100 g/l)
Primary Outcome/s	• **30-Day mortality**: No significant difference
Secondary Outcome/s	• **In-hospital mortality**: Significantly lower in the restrictive group • Subgroup analysis showed that restrictive transfusion notably improved survival in patients with lower illness severity (APACHE II ≤20) and those younger than 55, but it did not significantly benefit those with cardiac disease, severe infections or septic shock, and trauma. • **Cardiac events**: Significantly more common in the liberal group • **ICU mortality, 60-Day mortality**: No significant difference
Viva Summary	In a study involving critically ill patients with euvolaemia, a comparison was made between two approaches to red-cell transfusion thresholds: a restrictive threshold (Hb 70 g/l) and a liberal threshold (Hb 100 g/l). The primary outcome of 30-day mortality was not significantly different between the two groups. However, the restrictive group had lower in-hospital mortality, while the liberal group had a higher incidence of cardiac events. Subgroup analysis revealed that the restrictive transfusion strategy was particularly beneficial for patients with lower illness severity (APACHE II ≤20) and those younger than 55 years old, but it did not significantly benefit those with cardiac disease, severe infections or septic shock, or trauma.

(Continued)

(Continued)

Study Conclusion	'A restrictive strategy of red-cell transfusion is at least as effective as and possibly superior to a liberal transfusion strategy in critically ill patients, with the possible exception of patients with acute myocardial infarction and unstable angina.'

TRICC (1999): Hébert PC, Wells G, Blajchman MA, et al. A multicenter, randomized, controlled clinical trial of transfusion requirements in critical care. N Engl J Med. 1999;340(6):409–417.

Study Name	TRICS-III (2017)
Population	Patients undergoing cardiac surgery with EuroSCORE ≥1 (moderate to high risk of death)
Intervention	Restrictive red-cell transfusion threshold of 75 g/l vs liberal red-cell transfusion threshold of 95 g/l intra/post-op or 85 g/l on non-ICU ward
Primary Outcome/s	• **Day-28 or in-hospital composite of death, MI, New-onset AKI requiring dialysis**: A restrictive transfusion threshold was just as effective (non-inferior) as a liberal transfusion threshold
Secondary Outcome/s	• **LOS, Duration of ventilation, AKI, Seizures, Delirium**: No significant difference
Viva Summary	In a study involving cardiac surgery patients at moderate to high risk of death, a comparison was made between two red-cell transfusion thresholds: a restrictive threshold of 75 g/l and a liberal threshold of 95 g/l intra/post-op, or 85 g/l on non-ICU wards. The primary outcome, a composite of death, myocardial infarction, and new-onset acute kidney injury requiring dialysis within 28 days or during the hospital stay, showed that the restrictive threshold was just as effective as the liberal one (non-inferior). Secondary outcomes, including LOS, duration of ventilation, acute kidney injury, seizures, and delirium, were not significantly different between the two threshold groups.
Study Conclusion	'In patients undergoing cardiac surgery who were at moderate-to-high risk for death, a restrictive strategy regarding red-cell transfusion was noninferior to a liberal strategy with respect to the composite outcome of death from any cause, myocardial infarction, stroke, or new-onset renal failure with dialysis, with less blood transfused.'

TRICS-III (2017): Mazer CD, Whitlock RP, Fergusson DA, et al. Restrictive or liberal red-cell transfusion for cardiac surgery. N Engl J Med. 2017; 377(22):2133–2144.

PLATELET TRANSFUSIONS

Study Name	PACER (2023)
Population	Haematology or ICU patients with severe thrombocytopenia (platelet count 10,000–50,000 per mm³) undergoing CVC insertion
Intervention	Prophylactic platelet transfusion (1 unit) vs no platelet transfusion before CVC insertion

Primary Outcome/s	• **Incidence of grade 2–4 catheter-related bleeding within 24 hours**: Significantly lower in platelet transfusion group
	  – Grade 2: Required minor interventions e.g. >20 minutes of compression
	  – Grade 3: Required radiologic/elective intervention, or red cell transfusion
	  – Grade 4: Involved haemodynamic instability and increased transfusion, or death

Secondary Outcome/s	• **Platelet count at 1 hour and 24 hours, ICU LOS, Costs related to transfusion**: Significantly higher in transfusion group • **ICU/Hospital mortality, Risk of grade 3–4 catheter-related bleeding (more severe bleeding), Haematoma occurrence, Allergic transfusion reaction, Rate of red-cell transfusion within 24 hours**: No significant difference
Viva Summary	In a study involving haematology or ICU patients with severe thrombocytopenia (platelet count 10,000–50,000 per mm³) undergoing CVC insertion, a comparison was made between the effects of prophylactic platelet transfusion (1 unit) and no platelet transfusion before the procedure. The primary outcome measured was the incidence of grade 2–4 catheter-related bleeding within 24 hours, which was significantly lower in the platelet transfusion group. Secondary outcomes included platelet count at 1 hour and 24 hours, ICU LOS, and transfusion-related costs, all of which were significantly higher in the transfusion group. There were no significant differences in ICU/hospital mortality, risk of more severe catheter-related bleeding, haematoma occurrence, allergic transfusion reaction, or the rate of red-cell transfusion within 24 hours between the two groups.

Study Name	PACER (2023)
Study Conclusion	'The withholding of prophylactic platelet transfusion before CVC placement in patients with a platelet count of 10,000 to 50,000 per cubic millimeter did not meet the predefined margin for noninferiority and resulted in more CVC-related bleeding events than prophylactic platelet transfusion.'

PACER (2023): van Baarle FLF, van de Weerdt EK, van der Velden WJFM, et al. Platelet transfusion before CVC placement in patients with thrombocytopenia. N Engl J Med. 2023 May 25;388(21):1956–1965.

AGE OF CELLS FOR TRANSFUSION

Study Name	Zhang et al. (2019)
Population	Critically ill patients in ICU
Intervention	Fresh red-cell transfusion vs older red-cell transfusion (standard practice)
Primary Outcome/s	• **90-Day mortality**: No significant difference
Secondary Outcome/s	• **28/30-Day mortality, ICU/In-hospital mortality**: No significant difference
Viva Summary	In a study involving critically ill patients in the ICU, a comparison was made between fresh red-cell transfusions and older red-cell transfusions (standard practice). Ninety-day mortality was not significantly different between the two groups. Additionally, secondary outcomes, including 28/30-day mortality and ICU/in-hospital mortality, were not significantly different.
Study Conclusion	'The study concluded that age of red cells for transfusion did not affect the outcomes in critically ill patients.'

Zhang W, Yu K, Chen N, Chen M. Age of red cells for transfusion and outcomes in critically ill patients: a meta-analysis. Transfus Med Hemother. 2019 Aug;46(4):248–255.

SUMMARY

1. **TRICC (1999):** In a study involving critically ill patients with euvolaemia, a comparison was made between two approaches to red-cell transfusion thresholds: a restrictive threshold (Hb 70 g/l) and a liberal threshold (Hb 100 g/l). The primary outcome of 30-day mortality was not significantly different between the two groups. However, the restrictive group had lower in-hospital mortality, while the liberal group had a higher incidence of cardiac events. Subgroup analysis revealed that the restrictive transfusion strategy was particularly beneficial for patients with lower illness severity (APACHE II ≤20) and those younger than 55 years old, but it did not significantly benefit those with cardiac disease, severe infections or septic shock, or trauma.

2. **TRICS-III (2017):** In a study involving cardiac surgery patients at moderate to high risk of death, a comparison was made between two red-cell transfusion thresholds: a restrictive threshold of 75 g/l and a liberal threshold of 95 g/l intra/post-op, or 85 g/l on non-ICU wards. The primary outcome, a composite of death, myocardial infarction, and new-onset acute kidney injury requiring dialysis within 28 days or during the hospital stay, showed that the restrictive threshold was just as effective as the liberal one (non-inferior). Secondary outcomes, including LOS, duration of ventilation, acute kidney injury, seizures, and delirium, were not significantly different between the two threshold groups.

3. **PACER (2023):** In a study involving haematology or ICU patients with severe thrombocytopenia (platelet count 10,000–50,000 per mm³) undergoing CVC insertion, a comparison was made between the effects of prophylactic platelet transfusion (1 unit) and no platelet transfusion before the procedure. The primary outcome measured was the incidence of grade 2–4 catheter-related bleeding within 24 hours, which was significantly lower in the platelet transfusion group. Secondary outcomes included platelet count at 1 hour and 24 hours, ICU LOS, and transfusion-related costs, all of which were significantly higher in the transfusion group. There were no significant differences in ICU/hospital mortality, risk of more severe catheter-related bleeding, haematoma occurrence, allergic transfusion reaction, or the rate of red-cell transfusion within 24 hours between the two groups.

4. **Zhang et al. (2019):** In a study involving critically ill patients in the ICU, a comparison was made between fresh red-cell transfusions and older red-cell transfusions (standard practice). Ninety-day mortality was not significantly different between the two groups. Additionally, secondary outcomes, including 28/30-day mortality and ICU/in-hospital mortality, were not significantly different.

ANTIMICROBIAL THERAPY

Study Name	Wirz et al. (2018)
Population	Critically ill patients with sepsis of any type in the ICU
Intervention	Procalcitonin-guided antibiotic therapy vs standard care
Primary Outcome/s	• **Mortality within 30 days**: Significantly lower in procalcitonin-guided group
Secondary Outcome/s	• **Duration of antibiotic treatment**: Significantly earlier discontinuation of antibiotics in procalcitonin-guided group • **ICU/Hospital LOS**: No significant difference
Viva Summary	In a study involving critically ill sepsis patients in the ICU, a comparison was made between procalcitonin-guided antibiotic therapy and standard care. The procalcitonin-guided group exhibited a significantly lower 30-day mortality rate and discontinued antibiotics earlier, with no significant difference in ICU/hospital LOS between the two groups.
Study Conclusion	'Procalcitonin-guided antibiotic treatment in ICU patients with infection and sepsis patients results in improved survival and lower antibiotic treatment duration.'

Wirz Y, Meier MA, Bouadma L, et al. Effect of procalcitonin-guided antibiotic treatment on clinical outcomes in intensive care unit patients with infection and sepsis patients: a patient-level meta-analysis of randomized trials. Crit Care. 2018 Aug 15;22(1):191.

Study Name	CandiSep (2022)
Population	Septic adults at high risk for invasive *Candida* infection (ICI)
Intervention	(1,3)-β-D-glucan (BDG)–guided antifungal strategy vs standard treatment
Primary Outcome/s	• **28-Day mortality**: No significant difference
Secondary Outcome/s	• **Hospital mortality, Hospital/ICU LOS, VFDs, Vasopressor-free days, Cost**: No significant difference • **Percentage of patients receiving antifungals**: Significantly higher in BDG group • **Time to antifungal treatment**: Significantly shorter in BDG group
Viva Summary	In a study involving septic adults at high risk for ICI, BDG-guided antifungal strategy was compared to standard treatment. The primary outcome, 28-day mortality, was not significantly different between the two groups. Additionally, secondary outcomes, including hospital mortality, hospital/ICU LOS, VFDs, vasopressor-free days, and cost, were not significantly different. However, the percentage of patients receiving antifungal medication was significantly higher in the BDG group, and the time to antifungal treatment was significantly shorter in the BDG group.
Study Conclusion	'Serum BDG guided antifungal treatment did not improve 28-day mortality among sepsis patients with risk factors for but unexpected low rate of ICI. This study cannot comment on the potential benefit of BDG-guidance in a more selected at-risk population.'

CandiSep (2022): Bloos F, Held J, Kluge S, Simon P et al.; SepNet Study Group. (1→3)-β-D-Glucan-guided antifungal therapy in adults with sepsis: the CandiSep randomized clinical trial. Intensive Care Med. 2022 Jul;48(7): 865–875.

SUMMARY

1. **Wirz et al. (2018):** In a study involving critically ill sepsis patients in the ICU, a comparison was made between procalcitonin-guided antibiotic therapy and standard care. The procalcitonin-guided group exhibited a significantly lower 30-day mortality rate and discontinued antibiotics earlier, with no significant difference in ICU/hospital LOS between the two groups.

2. **CandiSep (2022):** In a study involving septic adults at high risk for invasive *Candida* infection, BDG-guided antifungal strategy was compared to standard treatment. The primary outcome, 28-day mortality, was not significantly different between the two groups. Additionally, secondary outcomes, including hospital mortality, hospital/ICU LOS, VFDs, vasopressor-free days, and cost, were not significantly different. However, the percentage of patients receiving antifungal medication was significantly higher in the BDG group, and the time to antifungal treatment was significantly shorter in the BDG group.

PREGNANCY AND POST-PARTUM

Study Name	Magpie (2002)
Population	Women with pre-eclampsia
Intervention	Magnesium sulphate vs placebo
Primary Outcome/s	• **Eclampsia**: Significantly lower with magnesium sulphate
Secondary Outcome/s	• **Maternal morbidity, Neonatal morbidity**: No significant difference (the only significant difference in morbidity was related to placental abruption) • **Side effects**: Significantly higher in magnesium group (e.g. flushing, nausea/vomiting, muscle weakness, headache, hypotension)
Viva Summary	In a study comparing magnesium sulphate to a placebo for women with pre-eclampsia, it was found that magnesium sulphate significantly reduced the occurrence of eclampsia. However, there was no significant difference in maternal and neonatal morbidity between the two groups, except for a higher incidence of side effects in the magnesium group, including flushing, nausea/vomiting, muscle weakness, headache, and hypotension.
Study Conclusion	'Magnesium sulphate halves the risk of eclampsia, and probably reduces the risk of maternal death. There do not appear to be substantive harmful effects to mother or baby in the short term.'

Magpie (2002): The Magpie Trial Collaborative Group. Do women with pre-eclampsia, and their babies, benefit from magnesium sulphate? The Magpie Trial: a randomised placebo-controlled trial. Lancet. 2002;359(9321):1877–1890.

DOI: 10.1201/9781003468738-8

Study Name	WOMAN (2017)
Population	Patients with post-partum haemorrhage (PPH)
Intervention	IV tranexamic acid (TXA) 1-g over 10 minutes vs placebo
Primary Outcome/s	• **Composite of 42-day all-cause mortality/hysterectomy**: No significant difference
Secondary Outcome/s	• **Death due to bleeding**: Significantly lower with TXA • **Thromboembolism**: No significant difference
Viva Summary	In a study involving patients with PPH, the comparison was made between the administration of 1-g of IV TXA over 10 minutes and placebo. The primary outcome, a composite of 42-day all-cause mortality and hysterectomy, was not significantly different between the two groups. However, secondary outcomes of death due to bleeding were significantly lower in the TXA group, while there was no significant difference in thromboembolism rates.
Study Conclusion	'Tranexamic acid reduces death due to bleeding in women with post-partum haemorrhage with no adverse effects. When used as a treatment for postpartum haemorrhage, tranexamic acid should be given as soon as possible after bleeding onset.'

WOMAN (2017): WOMAN Trial Collaborators. Effect of early tranexamic acid administration on mortality, hysterectomy, and other morbidities in women with post-partum haemorrhage (WOMAN): an international, randomised, double-blind, placebo- controlled trial. Lancet. 2017;389(10084):2105–2116.

Study Name	INTERCOVID (2021)
Population	COVID-19 in pregnancy (laboratory, radiological, or symptomatic diagnosis)
Interventions	None (observational study)
Key Findings	• A total of 8.4% of pregnant COVID-19 patients were admitted to critical care. • Higher risk of: 　• Pre-eclampsia/eclampsia 　• Severe infections 　• ICU admission 　• Maternal mortality 　• Preterm birth 　• Medically indicated preterm birth 　• Severe Neonatal Morbidity Index 　• Severe Perinatal Morbidity and Mortality Index • Fever and SOB were associated with a higher risk of severe maternal complications and neonatal complications • Asymptomatic COVID-19 in pregnancy was linked to a higher risk of maternal morbidity and pre-eclampsia
Viva Summary	In a study of pregnant women with COVID-19, 8.4% of patients required critical care. They had an increased risk of pre-eclampsia/eclampsia, severe infections, ICU admission, maternal mortality, preterm birth, medically indicated preterm birth, severe neonatal morbidity, and perinatal morbidity and mortality. Fever and shortness of breath were also associated with a higher risk of severe complications for both mothers and newborns, while asymptomatic COVID-19 during pregnancy was linked to a higher risk of maternal morbidity and pre-eclampsia.
Study Conclusion	'In this multinational cohort study, COVID-19 in pregnancy was associated with consistent and substantial increases in severe maternal morbidity and mortality and neonatal complications when pregnant women with and without COVID-19 diagnosis were compared. The findings should alert pregnant individuals and clinicians to implement strictly all the recommended COVID-19 preventive measures.'

INTERCOVID (2021): Villar J, Ariff S, Gunier RB, et al. Maternal and neonatal morbidity and mortality among pregnant women with and without COVID-19 infection: the INTERCOVID multinational cohort study. JAMA Pediatr. 2021;175(8):817–826.

SUMMARY

1. **Magpie (2002):** In a study comparing magnesium sulphate to a placebo for women with pre-eclampsia, it was found that magnesium sulphate significantly reduced the occurrence of eclampsia. However, there was no significant difference in maternal and neonatal morbidity between the two groups, except for a higher incidence of side effects in the magnesium group, including flushing, nausea/vomiting, muscle weakness, headache, and hypotension.

2. **WOMAN (2017):** In a study involving patients with PPH, the comparison was made between the administration of 1 g of IV TXA over 10 minutes and placebo. The primary outcome, a composite of 42-day all-cause mortality and hysterectomy, was not significantly different between the two groups. However, secondary outcomes of death due to bleeding were significantly lower in the TXA group, while there was no significant difference in thromboembolism rates.

3. **INTERCOVID (2021):** In a study of pregnant women with COVID-19, 8.4% of patients required critical care. They had an increased risk of pre-eclampsia/eclampsia, severe infections, ICU admission, maternal mortality, preterm birth, medically indicated preterm birth, severe neonatal morbidity, and perinatal morbidity and mortality. Fever and shortness of breath were also associated with a higher risk of severe complications for both mothers and newborns, while asymptomatic COVID-19 during pregnancy was linked to a higher risk of maternal morbidity and pre-eclampsia.

REHABILITATION AND FOLLOW-UP

Study Name	PRaCTICaL (2009)
Population	Patients aged >18 years discharged from ICU
Intervention	Nurse-led intensive care follow-up programmes vs standard care
Primary Outcome/s	• **Health-related quality of life at 12 months (using the SF-36 score):** No significant difference
Secondary Outcome/s	• **Cost:** Follow-up programmes were significantly more costly than standard care
Viva Summary	In a study involving adult patients discharged from the ICU, nurse-led intensive care follow-up programs were compared to standard care. The primary outcome of health-related quality of life at 12 months using the SF-36 score was not significantly different between the two groups. However, the follow-up programmes incurred significantly higher costs compared to standard care.
Study Conclusion	'A nurse led intensive care follow-up programme showed no evidence of being effective or cost effective in improving patients' quality of life in the year after discharge from intensive care. Further work should focus on the roles of early physical rehabilitation, delirium, cognitive dysfunction, and relatives in recovery from critical illness. Intensive care units should review their follow-up programmes in light of these results.'

PRaCTICaL (2009): Cuthbertson BH, Rattray J, Campbell MK, Gager M et al; PRaCTICaL Study Group. The PRaCTICaL study of nurse led, intensive care follow-up programmes for improving long term outcomes from critical illness: a pragmatic randomised controlled trial. BMJ. 2009 Oct 16;339:b3723.

DOI: 10.1201/9781003468738-9

Study Name	TEAM (2022)
Population	Mechanically ventilated adult patients in the ICU
Intervention	Early mobilisation (sedation minimisation and daily physiotherapy) vs standard care
Primary Outcome/s	• **Days alive and out of the hospital at day 180**: No significant difference
Secondary Outcome/s	• **Death at day 180, VFDs at day 28, ICU-free days at day 28, Functional outcome scores at day 180**: No significant difference • **Adverse events potentially due to mobilisation (arrhythmias, altered BP, desaturation)**: Significantly higher in early mobilisation group
Viva Summary	In a study involving mechanically ventilated adult ICU patients, a comparison was made between early mobilisation, which included sedation minimisation and daily physiotherapy, versus standard care. The number of days patients were alive and out of the hospital at day 180 was not significantly different between the two groups. Similarly, secondary outcomes including death at day 180, VFDs at day 28, ICU-free days at day 28, and functional outcome scores at day 180 did not significantly differ between the groups. However, the early mobilisation group did experience significantly higher rates of adverse events potentially related to mobilisation, such as arrhythmias, altered blood pressure, and desaturation.
Study Conclusion	'Among adults undergoing mechanical ventilation in the ICU, an increase in early active mobilization did not result in a significantly greater number of days that patients were alive and out of the hospital than did the usual level of mobilization in the ICU. The intervention was associated with increased adverse events.'

TEAM (2022): TEAM Study Investigators and the ANZICS Clinical Trials Group; Hodgson CL, Bailey M, Bellomo R, et al. Early active mobilization during mechanical ventilation in the ICU. N Engl J Med. 2022 Nov 10;387(19):1747–1758.

SUMMARY

1. **PRaCTICaL (2009):** In a study involving adult patients discharged from the ICU, nurse-led intensive care follow-up programmes were compared to standard care. The primary outcome of health-related quality of life at 12 months using the SF-36 score was not significantly different between the two groups. However, the follow-up programs incurred significantly higher costs compared to standard care.

2. **TEAM (2022):** In a study involving mechanically ventilated adult ICU patients, a comparison was made between early mobilisation, which included sedation minimisation and daily physiotherapy, versus standard care. The number of days patients were alive and out of the hospital at day 180 was not significantly different between the two groups. Similarly, secondary outcomes including death at day 180, VFDs at day 28, ICU-free days at day 28, and functional outcome scores at day 180 did not significantly differ between the groups. However, the early mobilisation group did experience significantly higher rates of adverse events potentially related to mobilisation, such as arrhythmias, altered blood pressure, and desaturation.

Printed in the United States
by Baker & Taylor Publisher Services

Printed in the United States
by Baker & Taylor Publisher Services